What the hell is wrong with me?

What the hell is wrong with me?

How to recover from pain, fatigue, weakness and other **undiagnosed** symptoms

Dr Gillian Deakin

'An extremely well-balanced and informed educational book. Easy to read and understand. Covering all functional information, this book is a must-read.'

Belinda, FND patient

'When your symptoms are real but elude conventional diagnosis, Dr Gillian Deakin redirects your search from the frustrating quest for answers to the emerging science of functional conditions, revealing that what is "wrong" with you may not be what you anticipate. Her unique mix of warmth, humour, and directness simplifies the complexities of undiagnosed symptoms, making them manageable and actionable. Her clear roadmap to recovery expertly guides you from uncertainty to confidently regaining your health.'

Sonja Armstrong, MSc (Nutrition & Functional Medicine)

'Dr Deakin finally lifts the veil on one of the most profound and little-known aspects of health which can severely and insidiously affect anyone's physical condition. Finally we are heard and understood. Thank you.'

Vero, FND patient

'Dr Deakin's book describes the complexities of so-called functional symptoms and conditions in a clear and easy-to-read form. It shines a light on what is an often misunderstood health problem. It gives hope and tools towards empowerment and improved health or recovery for patients struggling with these common and sometimes very disabling persistent symptoms. It is also an inspiration and guidance for clinicians as well as a good introduction to functional symptoms for students in the medical field.'

Anna-Karin Norlin, PhD, MD, specialist in general medicine

'It can be very demoralising to have symptoms that doctors can't explain or treat. Being told complicated symptoms like fatigue or pain are "are all in your head" is simply not helpful or fair. Yet one in ten of us will have these so called "functional symptoms" which are not linked to a clear disease pattern. Engaging with the health system for answers often leads to a medical merry-go-round. Put simply, medical professionals can sometimes be stumped when symptoms don't fit into a neat diagnosis. That is why Dr Gillian Deakin's book *What The Hell is Wrong With Me?* is so important and timely. Dr Deakin unpacks the complexity of just what functional symptoms are. As an outstanding science communicator, she takes us on a journey into the latest mind–body research which provides a framework for understanding and managing these complex symptoms. With great warmth, Dr Deakin gives voice to the many patients she has seen in her medical practice who share their stories, frustrations and hopes for the future.

'In a way, this book is like a toolkit for those who want insights and answers. It's for health professionals, patients and consumers who want to be able to understand and manage these symptoms more effectively. *What The Hell is Wrong With Me?* most importantly reassures anyone with functional symptoms that they are not alone.'

Dr Chris Cotton, GP

Acknowledgements

I am deeply grateful to the individuals whose support and expertise have been instrumental in bringing this book to fruition:

My friend and colleague, GP and health broadcaster, Dr Caroline West encouraged me to study clinical hypnotherapy, and it was a revelation to be able to temporarily induce symptoms such as numbness, paralysis, and loss of speech in otherwise healthy people. This phenomenon seemed similar to that in patients who were presenting with unexplained symptoms, and it set me on this journey of discovery for which I am deeply indebted to her.

Professor Kasia Kozlowska's groundbreaking research and pioneering treatments, generously shared in her open access book, helped reshape my understanding of functional conditions, allowing me to form the book's structure.

I sought the advice of Professor Peter Henningsen from the Clinic for Psychosomatic Medicine and Psychotherapy at the Technical University of Munich. He introduced me to the German national guidelines for the diagnosis and management of functional conditions, which were the result of his team's meticulous research efforts. His support has been vital in providing a structured approach to these often-confusing symptoms.

Flinders University's Speech therapy Professor Jan Baker's sage insights and clinical expertise and publications were instrumental in shaping the narrative of this book. Her support in introducing me to many others with expertise in this area has deepened my understanding of functional conditions.

Kate Faasse, Associate Professor of Health Psychology at the University of NSW, has contributed some brilliant work on the nocebo effect, which is necessary to understand functional conditions.

Yoga teacher Kay Parry and many others, too many to name, taught me the profound healing power of yoga as well as the need to persevere to attain its benefits.

I owe a great debt to the people who reviewed the manuscript and provided thoughtful, detailed suggestions:

Dr. Anna-Karin Norlin of the Pain and Rehabilitation Clinic, Linköping University, Sweden, has been of great assistance with her reading of the manuscript, endorsement, and thoughtful feedback. Her views were especially valued given her expertise in the management of functional conditions.

Occupational therapist Dr. Katherine Gill, founding director of FND Australia Support Services, provided invaluable assistance in recruiting many members who kindly read the manuscript and provided useful feedback.

Cardiologist and Professor of Medicine at Melbourne's Monash University, Dr. Murray Esler of the Baker Research Institute, generously shared his expertise in the Hypothalamic-Pituitary-Adrenal axis and the complexities of the physiological responses.

Neuropsychiatrist Dr. Adith Mohan and his team's innovative approach to patient care at the Neuropsychiatric Unit at Prince of Wales Hospital, Sydney, provided a useful perspective and inspiration that, with enough skill and determination, even quite unwell people can be provided with a means to manage their symptoms and lead better, more fulfilling lives.

Publishing director Ingrid Ohlsson provided timely guidance, helping me navigate the complex landscape of the publishing industry.

Bernadette Foley generously shared her extensive knowledge of the world of books, enriching the development of this project.

To all my patients, whose stories and experiences have served as the driving force behind this endeavour, I extend my deepest gratitude.

This production has relied on the expertise of Michael Hanrahan and his brilliant team at Publishing Central. Charlotte Duff's editing prowess is brilliant. It has been a joy to work with them.

Finally, to my family, for allowing the time and space throughout this journey.

First published in 2024 by Gillian Deakin

© Gillian Deakin 2024
The moral rights of the author have been asserted.

All rights reserved. Except as permitted under the *Australian Copyright Act 1968* (for example, a fair dealing for the purposes of study, research, criticism or review), no part of this book may be reproduced, stored in a retrieval system, communicated or transmitted in any form or by any means without prior written permission.

All inquiries should be made to the author.

ISBN: 978-1-923007-94-9

A catalogue entry for this book is available from the National Library of Australia.

Project management and text design by Publish Central
Cover design by Pipeline Design
Image page 61 © Shutterstock #93349765

Disclaimer: The material in this publication is of the nature of general comment only, and does not represent professional advice. It is not intended to provide specific guidance for particular circumstances and it should not be relied on as the basis for any decision to take action or not take action on any matter which it covers. Readers should obtain professional advice where appropriate, before making any such decision. To the maximum extent permitted by law, the author and associated entities and publisher disclaim all responsibility and liability to any person, arising directly or indirectly from any person taking or not taking action based on the information in this publication.

Contents

Introduction   1

Part I: Uncovering the basics of functional illness   9

Chapter 1	Functional illness: Facts and fiction	11
Chapter 2	What are functional symptoms?	23
Chapter 3	What causes functional illness?	35
Chapter 4	The seven stress response systems	45

Part II: Understanding pain, fatigue and the effect of negativity   77

Chapter 5	A kaleidoscope of pain in functional disorders	79
Chapter 6	Beyond exhaustion: Navigating the labyrinth of fatigue in functional disorders	99
Chapter 7	The nocebo effect and the surprising influence of negative thoughts	113
Chapter 8	Why the biomedical system is failing you – and where to turn to now	123

Part III: The path to recovery   139

Chapter 9	Step 1: Get a clear diagnosis	141
Chapter 10	Step 2: Shift the focus from treating the symptom to treating the cause	145
Chapter 11	Step 3: Identify which of your body stress systems are activated	153

Chapter 12	Step 4: Learn how to treat your functional condition	159
Chapter 13	Step 5: Build your team	165
Chapter 14	Step 6: Restore your seven body stress systems	181
Chapter 15	A few examples from each category to illustrate treatment options	209
Conclusion		217
Appendix A	Definitions	219
Appendix B	The seven body stress systems	225
Appendix C	Useful resources	229
Appendix D	Illness behaviour questionnaire	233
Index		237

Introduction

'It's all in your head!'
'Nothing is wrong with you.'
'It should just settle if you take it easy.'

Have you a bodily symptom that couldn't be explained by doctors? You've told your story (again!), been poked and prodded, gone through medical tests, seen specialists, yet no-one seems to have an answer. You've been told it's all in your head or that you should just take it easy, but that doesn't solve the problem.

And what do you do if the symptoms persist, or they come and go in a frightening manner, or they disrupt your day with their severity? What can help when your symptoms do not fit into a tidy medical diagnosis? Your symptoms are real and can be very disabling, but if no diagnosis has been made, how can you get treatment?

You are trying to live with an undiagnosed illness that has left you feeling frustrated, helpless and alone.

You're not alone. Look around. One person out of every 10 you see suffers from similar symptoms.[1]

The commonest condition you have never heard of

You might have pain or weakness. You might even have seizures, lose consciousness or be unable to speak. From the passing pain or

---

[1] Roenneberg C, Sattel H, Schaefert R, Henningsen P, Hausteiner-Wiehle C. Functional Somatic Symptoms. *Dtsch Arztebl Int*. 2019 Aug 9;116(33-34):553-560.

cough to the devastating collapse, things can happen in our bodies without any detectable disease. These symptoms have been called many things; we are now calling them 'functional'.

Functional symptoms are common. As a doctor with many years of experience, I see them all the time. While one in 10 people suffer from these symptoms, up to one in three patients seeing their GP have them! And I have seen functional disorders take many forms, from chronic pain to digestive issues, fatigue and headaches. Mercifully, many resolve quickly. But unfortunately, some can persist even for decades. If they are so common and sometimes so troubling, why is it so hard to get a clear diagnosis? What can be done to resolve these problems?

Let's take a closer look at these symptoms.

Everyone has had an odd symptom that seemed to come out of nowhere. We have all had a pain, a tic in the eyelid or a strange itch that came and went mysteriously. Maybe you nearly wet yourself or even worse? If you have had something weird happening in your body with no explanation, you may have had a 'functional' symptom.

Think of when you suddenly had abdominal pain or a wave of nausea. You didn't have an ongoing diagnosed problem such as an infection but nevertheless your symptom may have been as troublesome as it was unexplained.

Of greater concern are the sudden chest pains or faintness, shortness of breath or even difficulty walking. All these symptoms may be life-threatening or, at least, require urgent medical treatment – unless they are functional. How do you know and what should you do if you get some unexplained change in how your body functions?

This book is for all those who struggle with functional symptoms. You may have experienced these symptoms sporadically throughout your life, or they may have suddenly presented themselves. Regardless of how and when they started, you know they are real.

INTRODUCTION

Why I wrote this book

I have been studying and practising medicine for over 40 years and have seen many people like you, with symptoms that are not explained by any disease pattern.

Like you, I have been looking for answers to these unexplained symptoms and found very little in the standard medical texts and general literature, so I set out to use my research skills. I have been able to find some brilliant individuals, from within the medical profession and from a wide range of healers, all of whom have helped to shape my understanding of these perplexing health problems. This book is the result of a decades-long study.

After completing my degree at the University of Sydney, I practised medicine for a few years before commencing a doctoral degree on an Antarctic research station. On completing my thesis, I went on to study a master's degree in public health, which introduced me to many more ways to understand the causes of illness beyond just physical diseases – including the role of socioeconomic factors, environmental hazards, cultural determinants and psychological elements, which can all lead to changes in health, for better or worse.

When I eventually entered general practice, I found that many of my patients had health problems that were, at least in part, caused by factors beyond simply a medical disease. I have also worked in many different practices and noticed the level of health standards varied enormously depending on privilege. But even within very wealthy areas, such as Eastern Sydney, there remains a level of poor health that cannot be attributed to any physical disease, or environmental or social disadvantage, but nevertheless can have devastating effects on the lives of my patients.

This observation, that illness is not just a product of disease but many other factors, sent me on a search through other forms of health practices.

I was very fortunate to have grown up in a family who, in the 1960s, embraced a healthy lifestyle. So I have a lived experience of the benefits of a healthy diet, daily physical activity and spiritual wellbeing. At six, I thought having a cold shower was a normal part of your day!

Studying medicine, I was surprised to find so little emphasis on health, and I have gone on to learn more about how to enhance human wellbeing and resilience. I have been practising yoga now for 50 years and find its therapeutic benefits invaluable, both personally and for my patients.

I have also studied, practised and taught meditation, and have observed the profound shifts in individuals who embrace meditation in their lives.

Finally, I have learnt to use hypnotherapy and have a deeper understanding of how the subconscious parts of our minds can affect our state. This fascinating journey never ceases to amaze.

Continuing to seek ways to understand the development of functional symptoms, I finally came across the work of Dr Kasia Kozlowska and her colleagues at the Mind-Body Program at Westmead Hospital in Sydney. Her research into the body stress systems has been a vital contribution to our understanding of how the body responds to the infinite number of stresses we experience. Dr Kasia Kozlowska and her team have also worked with authorities from around the world to develop a sound, tried and tested approach to the treatment of functional conditions. While their focus is on children and adolescents, many of their formulations and approaches can be generalised to the adult population. This book is an attempt to bring her unit's methods to the broader public.

I have also utilised the excellent clinical guidelines on functional somatic symptoms issued by the German Association of Scientific Medical Societies (AWMF). These highly researched guidelines are excellent in that they embrace all bodily systems and are of direct practical use.

By collaborating with experts in the field of functional medicine from around the world, I have worked to develop a clear way to describe what has happened in your body and what to do about it.

The research into this new understanding is far from complete and the description given to you here is a simplified version of what the experts in the field are agreeing upon.

But the main source of my understanding has come through the generosity of my patients. In sharing their journey, they have helped me learn what led them to be sick and what aided their recovery. Their (de-identified) stories are used throughout this book to illustrate the role of the body stress systems in causing illness, and how we worked towards their recovery.

How to use this book

Medical science has made extraordinary advances over the last century and can help diagnose conditions with amazing precision, right down to the genetic cause.

But our current medical training generally does not equip us to help you deal with a condition when the history is unclear, examination reveals no concerns, and all tests are normal. You can be sent from doctor to doctor, from test to test, all to no avail. You may be putting up with costly and time-consuming assessments on top of nasty, distressing symptoms, and yet you are no closer to getting relief – until now.

It can be very frustrating to have symptoms that nobody can explain or treat. But the good news is these symptoms are becoming less of a puzzle.

At last, doctors and researchers around the world are finally gaining some understanding of what causes these mysterious symptoms and, better still, how to treat them – and I include these new understandings and findings in this book.

I share with you:
- what you need to know about your symptoms and many others
- the factors that come together to cause these symptoms
- how to resolve your symptoms.

I delve into your amazing body stress systems, outlining how they both protect you, but also can become disrupted. In the chapters in part I of this book, I cover the basics of these functional symptoms – including explaining the use of the term 'functional'. In part II, we explore the causes of pain and fatigue much more deeply, and I highlight the importance of the brain–body connection, as well as how modern medicine may be failing you. In part III, we get to the chapters you're likely most interested in, covering the path to recovery, the different ways to restore function, and how you can work through the six steps with your healthcare team to get the care you need.

A word of warning, though – don't be tempted to jump straight to the chapters in part III. You first need to read the earlier chapters to understand the important foundations underlying this treatment approach. Without this understanding, the chapters in part III won't make sense.

I've also included a glossary of terms and other helpful resources in the appendices. And, to help you understand your condition more fully and see you are far from alone, throughout the book I use stories like Madeline's.

MADELINE

'I've got so many things wrong with me, I don't know where to begin,' Madeline gushed as soon as she sat down. She started to list her symptoms and I could see straightaway that this was no ordinary illness: sore throat, rashes, upset gut. Worst of all, her fatigue prevented her from doing her work.

As we tried to sort out the history of each symptom, Madeline struggled to give a clear account. The symptoms were intermittent and seemed not to follow any pattern. She had seen other doctors and had a swag of tests, but nothing could explain her perplexing and debilitating symptoms. What on earth could cause all these problems and yet show no signs of disease in any test?

> Madeline's story is unique, but her illness was eventually diagnosed. Over a period, we were able to establish that Madeline's symptoms were functional and, once this was understood and accepted by both her doctor and herself, and the right treatment was commenced, she steadily recovered.
>
> People with health problems like Madeline's often seek to get treated in the same way she did, as if expecting a simple physical diagnosis. She had test after test, but none of them suggested anything was wrong with her. Many people like Madeline have never heard about functional conditions, and it is time that changed.

Some people simply have no explanation for their symptoms and the best we can offer them is recognition and support. Linus is an example of this.

> **LINUS**
> Linus is a delightful, quirky individual who has had a number of interesting medical conditions over the years. These conditions have been diagnosed and treated so he remains extremely well, now doing volunteer work as well as travelling around the country for his job. However, about 10 years ago, he developed a pain between his eyes. We checked everything and he has seen a number of specialists over the years, but no-one can solve the mystery. Linus is remarkable in his stoicism. We both agree that focusing on others may be his best way of coping. His volunteer work is a helpful distraction.

There are thousands of people like Linus, and the medical profession simply has nothing to offer them. This book is for those who, like the other cases throughout this book, can use a model of care that is often effective to treat their symptoms.

In this book, we will uncover the many potential causes of functional symptoms, including biological, nutritional, genetic, epigenetic, psychological, immunological, social, and environmental factors. Together, we will delve into the latest research and break down the key concepts you need to know to better understand your condition.

This book will provide you with the tools to understand and manage your functional symptoms effectively. You will learn how to apply this radical approach and begin to heal yourself. Tried and tested again and again, we now have the means to treat some of the most debilitating symptoms. In one study, simply the explanation of the cause of the symptoms was enough to resolve the symptoms in 27 per cent of the patients!

I hope that you will find these approaches helpful and that, through education, you can be empowered to take control of your health and ultimately improve your quality of life.

So let's begin.

Part I: Uncovering the basics of functional illness

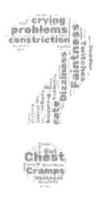

Chapter 1

Functional illness: Facts and fiction

Over the centuries, many terms have been used to describe your symptoms but, even now, doctors and researchers still can't agree on a term to define them. Adding to this confusion are a whole lot of alternate practitioners, each with their own notion about what is affecting you. And then there's the internet with its 'diagnosis by algorithm'. Perhaps you've even heard of (or received) the vague diagnosis of 'medically unexplained symptoms'.

> The reason that the term 'medically unexplained symptoms' has largely been abandoned is that your symptoms usually can be explained, with enough time and effort.

While agreeing that there is no perfect term, what many doctors have settled on – and what I use in this book – is 'functional symptoms'. Each term has its uses and limitations, and even the term 'functional' is initially confusing, but the following definition will help to explain it: Functional conditions or functional somatic[2] symptoms are a *disturbance* of normal functioning of bodily processes; these occur in a body when all the usual tests of the body appear normal, and the body 'misbehaves' or 'malfunctions'.

But what exactly does this mean? Let's look at some of the facts – and fictions – about functional conditions.

A glitch in your software

Comparing your body to a computer might help you get your head around functional symptoms: physical disorders are like having a hardware problem, whereas functional disorders are like a software problem. You don't need to keep checking the hardware. Your 'hardware' – that is, your body – is fine.

But several factors have led to a disruption in the software – in other words, in the *functioning* of your body. Your body systems and interconnecting neural network (brain, spine and nerves) have become temporarily disrupted, which is why you have these symptoms.

In this book, I take you through a radical, new approach to your symptoms that will help you to focus on reprogramming your 'software' to restore normal functioning. We will explore what your 'software' is and why it got disrupted.

One thing that most doctors agree on is that treating patients with these diagnoses is challenging because their medical training does not equip them to deal with functional conditions.

It is vital to state at the outset that no one doctor, healer, belief system, test or treatment can easily treat the vast array of symptoms that arise through this disruption. I often work with other health practitioners to find the best way forward. We still have a lot to learn about functional disorders and not all experts agree on the best approach, so if you have found a useful means to understand your condition, and have recovered, you are fortunate. But, given

---

[2] Somatic means relating to the body, as opposed to mental or psychological symptoms.

the complex causes of functional conditions, your solution may not apply to others. As journalist and essayist HL Mencken noted, 'For every complex problem there is an answer that is clear, simple, and wrong.'

If you have ongoing symptoms, you may be discovering that functional conditions are hard to understand and easy to misunderstand. They are difficult both to explain and to treat, especially in the usual health setting of a quick visit to the doctor or the emergency department. You may have found that your medical team have been unhelpful, and you have been discharged without any clear diagnosis or advice on what to do. But in this book, we will explore what experts now know about functional conditions and what you can do to recover from them.

Not faked, not imagined

Malingering – that is, feigning sickness or injury – does occur, of course, but it is much rarer and not the subject of this book. Your symptoms are just as real as they would be if you did have a known physical condition or medically recognised disease. This is why you may believe that you do have a physical disease. You did not cause your symptoms, and there are things you can do to help them go away.

> If you are living with a functional condition, your symptoms are not imagined. They are not 'just in your head'.

Your doctor has likely done tests that ruled out pathology in your body. So, if the cause of your symptoms is not 'just in your head' and it's not in your body, where the hell is it? Read on!

When doctors run tests, they test your anatomy for signs of disease and they test your chemistry for imbalances or deficiencies.

What they may miss in these tests are the changes in your physiology – that is, how your body functions – which are causing your symptoms. The reason for this is that they assume that any changes in your physiology will correct themselves, because that is usually what happens. We now know that if you have a persistent functional symptom, your physiology has not returned your body back to its usual operating mode.

For example, everyone has experienced a tingling sensation through their body – such as when a child runs in front of their car. But Jonas reported that this was happening to him intermittently for days at a time, with no obvious cause.

If you have functional symptoms, you have disruptions in one or more of your seven body stress systems. Every doctor knows about these systems, but it has been difficult to find an easy-to-understand way to explain how their disruption can cause your symptoms – until now. When I read the work of Australian psychiatrist Dr Kasia Kozlowska describing these body stress systems and how they can cause functional symptoms, I recognised how we can bridge the gap between the complex science and a common understanding of functional medicine.

The most misunderstood problem in the world of medicine

Approximately a third of patients who consult their doctor with physical symptoms have no standard medical explanation for those symptoms.[3] Mercifully, many of these symptoms are short-lived and settle without any need for intervention. But in a third of these people, the symptoms can persist for months or years and, without proper management, can cause disability, distress and prolonged illness behaviour – including absenteeism, anxiety, multiple medical

---

[3] Roenneberg C, Sattel H, Schaefert R, Henningsen P, Hausteiner-Wiehle C. Functional Somatic Symptoms. *Dtsch Arztebl Int*. 2019 Aug 9;116(33-34):553-560.

tests and interventions, severe suffering, and reduced quality of life (although, a functional condition usually won't shorten your life).

Unfortunately, a lot of doctors find it very difficult to know what to do when they can't find a physical disorder to explain the symptoms. They were not trained to recognise, let alone treat, these conditions.

And the bafflement may get translated into annoyance or other forms of dismissive treatment, and you may be treated with less than the usual respect you would receive if you were diagnosed with a physical complaint. Doctors are often as frustrated as you are. The diagnosis of a functional condition often creates negative feelings of doubt about the condition, fear on the part of the doctor that they might be missing something, annoyance that you continue to complain of something, even though all the tests suggest that you have a seemingly healthy body, and a feeling of inadequacy that they can't seem to help. It is not surprising that you may sense some of these feelings.

Given the vague outcome and seeming lack of treatment options, your feelings of confusion, as well as your expectation of a physical explanation for your symptoms, may be combined with fear that something has been overlooked, or the tests are inaccurate or a mistake has occurred somewhere along the way. With all the tests being normal, your doctor has no way of proving that your body is just producing symptoms without any evidence of disease. Understandably, you might feel angry that no-one is taking your symptoms seriously or you might feel dismissed.

What is worse is that your symptoms may persist *because* there seems to be no obvious treatment for them. This might lead to a state of hopelessness and helplessness. Unfortunately, the stress caused by this response will further activate your body stress systems and a vicious cycle can ensue. The worse your situation and your stressors, the worse your symptoms become.

The good news is that help is here. As you read through the chapters in this book, you will be brought up to date with the latest science and discover what we now know, and don't know, about functional conditions. And, by the end of this book, you will be on the path to healing.

The Bermuda Triangle of medicine

It may help to know that having a functional symptom places you in what we could call the Bermuda Triangle of medicine. Your symptoms (and you) simply do not register on the medical radar. You disappear from the screens of physical medicine once all the possible physical diseases have been ruled out. Since your symptoms have no physical cause, doctors tend to assume, wrongly, that they are entirely 'psychosomatic' (that is, caused or aggravated by a mental factor) and, therefore usually, not worthy of treatment by orthodox doctors. Perhaps you have been sent off to a psychiatrist.[4]

But you know that your symptoms *are* physical – your pain is real or you truly feel very dizzy or faint. So where should you go for help?

And how did this unsatisfactory healthcare system arise?

A brief history of illness

Whatever culture or historical period you live in, your symptoms are interpreted within the cultural constructs of the day. If you had been living before the scientific era – say, in Mediaeval Europe – you might have been told that a witch had cast an evil spell on you, or a disease-bearing wind was blowing. In traditional Chinese medicine, an imbalance of your yin and yang energy may be said to be the cause of illness. Hippocrates is said to have described the 'four humours' and this model of health and disease persisted until the modern era. The shamans, healers and physicians of the time were sought to explain all symptoms in terms acceptable to their

---

[4] Note that psychiatrists can be helpful with functional conditions but only after a full assessment of all possible factors, and once you agree that your mental health may play a contributing role.

community. So, whether you had a physical or functional symptom, you would be treated regardless.

But by the late nineteenth century, physicians were able to utilise the microscope and begin to measure vital signs. Illness stopped being *interpreted* by the physician. Doctors were able to record objective features of disease and measure changes – for example, in the blood. So, for over a hundred years, doctors have relied on tests rather than a broader understanding of the functioning of the human body. It is not surprising that functional symptoms have become a riddle wrapped in a mystery inside an enigma (with apologies to Churchill).

Nowadays, we have sophisticated instruments and tests to identify diseases. Only with such scientific testing did doctors begin to distinguish between 'medically explained' and 'functional' symptoms.

While many functional symptoms require tests to prove they are not due to a physical disease, sometimes simply your story is enough to clinch the diagnosis. Sachen was an example of this.

> **SACHEN**
> Sachen came to report a curious rash that occurred shortly after waking and would clear every night. He accepted that no medical condition causes such a pattern and he recognised the role of numerous life demands that had accumulated, and so undertook to reduce the burdens on him.

When the history or tests exclude every known problem with the physical body, then the doctor will determine that the illness suffered by the patient is not due to disease in a specific organ (such as the brain, stomach or heart), but rather due to a disturbance in the function of the otherwise healthy organ. This is why today the preferred term for medically unexplained symptoms is 'functional'. Through this book, I refer to functional symptoms, functional disorders and sometimes disorders specific to a bodily symptom, such as functional neurological disorders.

In chapter 8, I delve more deeply into how our understanding of illness has changed over the centuries and how our modern beliefs are causing problems for those with functional conditions.

Towards a medical understanding of your condition

You may have found your doctor has not given you a diagnosis. That is because they often were not taught about functional conditions in a systematic way. While functional disorders are beginning to be categorised and grouped in a way that will allow your doctor to treat you in the usual systematic fashion used with physical conditions, we still have a long way to go.

Doctors are skilled in the diagnosis of physical conditions but less confident about affirming something is functional. When a doctor makes a physical diagnosis – say, a heart attack – they need to have firm, scientific, verifiable evidence. This might include changes in the electrocardiogram (ECG) and blood tests that meet the well-established criteria for diagnosis. Here is medical science at its best.

The problem with functional symptoms is that diagnosing them relies on the tests being normal – that is, you go to the doctor with chest pain, and a normal ECG and blood test suggest you are not having a heart attack. But normal tests can't prove you are experiencing functional pain – for example, from the chest wall muscles. Understandably, you would likely think that if enough tests are done, a physical cause for your pain will emerge. And, of course, other causes of chest pain do exist. Emergency departments have protocols to rapidly identify the serious problems that require hospital treatment, such as heart attack or pulmonary embolism. But the diagnosis of complex and usually harmless, albeit distressing, conditions is not their responsibility.

Typically, if you went to hospital with chest pain due to a functional condition, the pain would settle and you would be sent away 'better'. But nothing has been proven and no definite diagnosis has been made. Other non-fatal causes of chest pain, such as shingles or severe reflux, would emerge over the following days and could be treated by your GP. If no further symptoms arose, the matter is usually laid to rest with the 'wait and see' approach, on the loose assumption that your pain may have been functional. Doctors are trained to hold several ideas at once and would be on the lookout for other possibilities.

But the diagnosis of a functional symptom can be difficult to accept for both you and your doctor. This is because of the scientific principle that the burden of proof lies with the one making the claim – if a doctor determines a symptom is functional, they need to be able to prove this claim. Because all the tests are normal with functional conditions, this does not prove anything – it only proves what the pain is *not* due to. This diagnostic vacuum is a very uncomfortable place for the scientifically minded.

If you have experienced the very real and frightening experience of chest pain, seeking a solid, verifiable diagnosis is totally understandable. It is very hard to believe that something so painful could be due to 'nothing'.

> Science here is a victim of its own success.
> Our society has come to expect a scientific answer for everything.

Now, many people feel that if a clear physical diagnosis to explain their symptoms is not forthcoming, someone has not done their job, particularly if the symptoms are novel or severe.

It's time that doctors and patients alike come to a healthier understanding of functional conditions:

- They can be severe or sudden.

- They can often appear out of the blue.
- They can have many causes, or no obvious cause.

In chapter 3, I explore the current understanding of the causes of functional symptoms in more detail, and how they are perceived by the brain.

Why is a diagnosis so important?

When a patient brings their symptoms to a doctor, they are seeking a way to understand their experience. When the doctor gives a name to their condition – that is, a diagnosis – they give validity and meaning to the patient's situation. The patient can externalise their symptoms, and they can depersonalise them. This makes their symptoms containable and manageable.

In contrast, when the tests fail to reveal a specific diagnosis, the patient is left with the unsettling knowledge that they are on their own with their collection of symptoms. No diagnosis is forthcoming, so no path forward can be given by the doctor. The patient is left in a quagmire of unclear and unorganised feelings, with no system of diagnosis to provide therapeutic direction.

> Without a diagnosis, your condition is boundless, anarchic and unpredictable. And no-one can tell you what will help. This is an incredibly difficult spot to find yourself.

At last, a diagnosis! But what now?

Fortunately, expert understanding of your condition has advanced and a diagnosis can and should be given to you, along with treatment, as I outline in the later chapters in this book. Research is revealing how the unique neural pathways in your brain and body might respond to various stressors. Be prepared to be surprised and challenged. But, mainly, be ready to find a path to better health and maybe even recovery.

One word of warning: be careful of labels that imply you are sicker than you are. If you are told, for example, that you have chronic fatigue syndrome, your likely next step is to google the condition and its symptoms. You might read that 'chronic' means lasting years or even a lifetime. This could be devastating and undermine your hopes for recovery. Only accept a label that serves to help your recovery.

So, if we are willing to accept the idea that functional conditions do exist, the next questions are what exactly are functional conditions and what could be causing them? In the following two chapters, I explore what is known so far about functional symptoms and their causes.

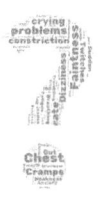

Chapter 2

What are functional symptoms?

We all have functional symptoms every day that are normal, purposeful reactions. That is, our body responds to our environment and our conscious and subconscious brain throughout the day and night. If you are cold, your body stress system responds by creating goose bumps. Our emotions and feelings also get expressed through bodily symptoms: laughing, crying and shaking with fear are a few examples of functional somatic expressions. I explore the full complexity of your body stress systems in chapter 4 but, for now, it helps to know that you get symptoms because your body stress systems have been activated.

Functional symptoms: what are they and who gets them?

Some functional symptoms are easy to connect with their psychological cause. For example, sadness will cause tears to flow. But some somatic responses seem to arise spontaneously and without any obvious cause. Waking up with chest pain should prompt immediate medical attention, but when the doctors rule out medical causes, it still can be difficult to recognise all factors that might lead to pain happening. Perhaps your mind is so fixated on a life problem that it is not aware of the stressors that the problem is generating. Or perhaps not. We just don't know.

Any new and troubling symptom warrants a proper diagnosis, and your doctor should take a careful history and complete an examination of your body to determine the cause of any symptoms, because two out of three patients who present to their general practitioner turn out to have a physical condition. But, as mentioned in the introduction, this means you have about one chance in three of having a functional cause for your symptom. Your body is simply not responding in the way you expect.

Functional symptoms can range from the trivial and commonplace, such as nervous cough or fleeting flutters (like 'butterflies' in the stomach) all the way through to severe, agonising pain, and complete system shutdown, such as total numbness, blindness, seizures or unconsciousness. They can be associated with strong emotions or no obvious psychological stress. They can be very brief, intermittent or persistent. They can last seconds or years. They can change from one side of the body to the other, from the top to the bottom, from the front to the back. They can be associated with other symptoms, such as nausea, sweating, dizziness, faintness, heaviness or inability to move. Whatever the symptoms, they share a similar origin. So, it is important to keep your focus on the causes and, yes, pay less heed to your symptom expression. I explain why in chapter 3.

Functional symptoms are common. They can also be contagious. It's difficult to see someone laughing without feeling the same urge to laugh. How long can you watch someone scratching before the sensation of an itch arises? And the larger the crowd reaction, the more contagious it can be.

Mass reactions occur particularly among social groupings that experience emotional and behavioural repression, such as what was expected from young women in the early 1960s. 'Beatlemania' was the term given to large groups of mainly young women who screamed, shook, fainted and even wet themselves, in response to being near their idols, The Beatles.

Functional symptoms are not unique to the modern era, either. Descriptions can be found in recorded history and in all cultures. (I explore the evolution and cultural interpretations of functional symptoms in chapter 8.)

> **TENSION HEADACHES: GATEWAY TO UNDERSTANDING FUNCTIONAL CONDITIONS**
>
> No doubt you've experienced a headache. One minute you are perfectly well, but then you start to develop some tightness or pressure and, before you know it, you have a full headache.
>
> After rest and maybe medication, you recover to your full health.
>
> Just like with all functional disorders, any blood tests and brain scans undertaken while you're experiencing this headache would be normal.
>
> But, of course, not only are the symptoms painfully real, but certain tests would be able to detect physiological changes in the body – for example, a tightening of the muscles of your head or neck.
>
> So, if you are a headache sufferer, you have a very real, and at times disabling, malady, but your tests are totally fine, and you make a full recovery after each headache. Unlike a headache due to, for example, meningitis, your tension headache is functional – with real symptoms and normal tests.
>
> Like other functional conditions, many factors can lead to a headache, with psychological stress being only one of them. Other stressors that can trigger the headache include:
>
> - dehydration
> - poor posture
> - overuse and tightness of muscles
> - nocturnal teeth grinding
> - certain work activities
> - frequent texting with head down, causing strain on neck muscles
> - crying a lot.

> Of course, if the onset of a headache triggers concerns of something serious developing, this will add to the stress burden.
> This holds true for nearly all functional conditions.
> Many headache sufferers know from experience that drinking more water and taking a break from slouching in front of a screen can help reduce headache frequency. So, searching for *all* the factors that cause your problem is an important part of the treatment of functional conditions.

Possible functional symptoms

I've provided in this section an incomplete list of symptoms that might be functional. Of course, they all could be due to a disease process, so it is important to make sure your doctor has ruled out physical disease before assuming these symptoms are functional. And when it comes to serious symptoms such as chest pain, especially if the pain persists for minutes, prompt action may save your life. It is not a good time to wonder if a body stress system is causing you to develop chest pain. Just call an ambulance.

Functional symptoms can include the following:

- a feeling of constriction in the chest
- a strong feeling of dread, danger or foreboding
- accelerated heart rate
- 'air hunger' (the feeling like you can't get enough breath), breathing difficulties, shortness of breath
- anxious and irrational thinking
- back pain
- blushing
- constipation
- double vision
- dry mouth
- dry, irritated eyes
- dyspepsia (indigestion)
- erectile dysfunction

- eye strain, fatigue
- faecal incontinence
- faintness
- fatigue, weakness
- fear of going mad, losing control or dying
- feelings of unreality, brain fog, dizziness, full loss of consciousness, light-headedness
- gait disturbance
- gut disturbances, nausea, abdominal distress or pain
- heightened vigilance for danger and physical symptoms
- hoarseness, change in pitch or volume of your speech
- hot flushes or cold chills
- hyperhidrosis (excessive sweating)
- incontinence
- irritable bowel syndrome
- joint and muscle pain
- loss of vision
- lump in the throat or feeling something stuck there
- not being able to urinate if anyone is around
- sudden emotional outburst (for example, crying)
- swallowing disorders
- sweating
- swelling, rashes and inflammation itch
- tense muscles, cramps, twitches, fleeting pains
- tingling, particularly in the arms and hands, numbness
- tinnitus or a buzzing/ringing sound
- trembling or shaking
- tunnel vision
- urinary frequency, burning, pain, urgency
- visual problems.

As you can see from this long but far from complete list of functional symptoms, several observations can be made:

- We all get some of these symptoms – whether it is some eye strain after a long day or a dry mouth when experiencing

unaccustomed social pressure – but usually they quickly resolve. We can understand their cause and can safely ignore them, knowing they will resolve when the situation changes.
- Nearly any bodily experience could be a functional response, a glitch in the system. Functional symptoms are experienced in the same way that symptoms due to physical causes are experienced, but there is no sign of disease.

In this book, I use three categories, (symptoms, syndromes and disorders), which describe the degree of impact of your symptoms.[5] Each category requires more levels of treatment added to the previous, as follows:

1. *Persistent functional **symptoms***: Ongoing non-specific symptoms that are burdensome enough for the patient to consult a doctor but are not classified as disease. If you have one of these symptoms, it may impair how you function daily. This might be a single symptom, such as a tic or a cough, that does not fit into a medical diagnosis.
2. *Functional somatic **syndromes***: If you have a defined symptom cluster, such as fibromyalgia syndrome or irritable bowel syndrome, you may have a greater disruption to everyday functioning. These syndromes are better described and have agreed management guidelines. Other examples include persistent fatigue and complex regional pain syndrome.
3. *Somatic stress **disorders***: If you have one of these disorders, life is very difficult because they are the most serious and disabling and are also associated with multiple symptoms that can affect your mood and your behaviour. Because your condition is often unique, you require a tailored treatment plan that you work on together with your healthcare team.

---

5   These categories are based on those found in Roenneberg, C, Sattel, H, Schaefert, R, Henningsen, P, Hausteiner-Wiehle, C (2019), 'Functional somatic symptoms', *Dtsch Arztebl Int*, Aug 9;116(33–34):553–560.

These conditions overlap and you may have more than one of them. They also occur with other conditions, including mental health problems in about 50 per cent of cases. In other words, diagnosis and treatment are complex.

For the remainder of this chapter, I've included a few stories about some of my patients with functional conditions, to give you a better idea of how these conditions can present quite differently. While acknowledging the uniqueness of each case, however, perhaps you will also see some similarities with your own experiences.

CARMEN

Carmen is a vibrant and energetic woman but she often attended with a litany of symptoms, including chest tightness, headaches, reflux, and back and shoulder aches. It was difficult to keep track of them all. She saw naturopaths, chiropractors and osteopaths. She had intravenous vitamin C too, but none of the efforts to cure her had any lasting effect. It was only after her once terrifyingly unpredictable mother died that Carmen felt able to reveal the extent of her childhood abuses. Gradually, with the support of ongoing trauma therapy, along with physical 'reprogramming' from her physiotherapist, the symptoms abated.

Carmen's persistent functional symptoms may have been partly due to her childhood experiences. A history of trauma is not uncommon among people with ongoing functional symptoms. (The reason for this will be elaborated in chapter 5.)

But most patients with functional conditions have not experienced severe trauma and abuse. Their life experiences might be quite commonplace.

MIN

Min is a hardworking nurse and mother of two young children. She rarely attended the practice but recently had become worried. She had been waking with the uncomfortable sensation of a lump or obstruction in the throat. After a proper assessment and tests, she was told that it was a functional condition called globus[6] and she was given some ways to manage the condition. Min found this far from satisfactory and wanted a second opinion. Her uncle had recently died from throat cancer and she was not convinced that her symptoms were nothing to worry about. Her symptoms took on a frightening significance and she couldn't focus on much else. Her sleep was affected and her family became fed up with her obsession.

Min needed repeated tests and a lot of education and assurance before she could accept a referral to a speech therapist who explained carefully to Min how the sensation of globus can arise. Sometimes, it can arise in association with reflux or other structural issues (which, in Min's case, had been explored and ruled out). More often than not, the sensation is in response to muscles of the larynx and throat becoming tight – especially if the person had been under a lot of pressure, possibly worrying about things, or dealing with feelings of sadness or worry that had been difficult to talk about. (I provide much more detail on these underlying causes in the chapters in part III.)

MICHAEL

At 35, Michael seemed to have it all: he was a tall, good-looking man, married to a lovely woman with one child and another on the way, and his career was flourishing. He had achieved many of his life goals. But his days were marred by the pain and misery of abdominal cramps, bloating and irregular bowel actions. After these symptoms had been fully investigated, Michael was told by the specialist that he had irritable bowel syndrome.

Irritable bowel syndrome is included in the second category from those listed earlier in this chapter – functional somatic

---

6 'Globus' is the name given to a feeling like there is a lump in the throat or something stuck there. The English language has a lot of expressions to describe this psychosomatic response: 'She gulped', 'He swallowed hard', 'Her throat constricted with fear', 'I felt choked up'. All these expressions are ways to describe globus, which occurs when the throat muscles tighten. It is an unpleasant if harmless sensation. But a feeling like the throat is about to close or become obstructed can be very frightening. A careful examination is required to ensure that there truly is no obstruction. Then attention should be given to all the factors that can lead to the globus occurring.

syndromes. These are better defined and recognised, with international agreements on the symptoms and findings necessary for diagnosis.

While all tests, including colonoscopy, are normal with this syndrome, physical symptoms are frequently very uncomfortable and sometimes the pain is severe enough to warrant a trip to hospital. And yet the body is otherwise perfectly healthy. This is a frustrating condition, where the various medications and diets only provide limited relief.

One day, Michael revealed that behind his calm demeanour, he struggled with anxiety, always fearing the judgement of others, and never feeling satisfied with his achievements. Worse yet, his mood disorder, which he had skilfully masked, was preventing him from connecting to his daughter. This caused him further distress, and his bowels 'went crazy'. He agreed to undergo psychotherapy and started some medication that eased both his anxiety and, to his great relief, much of his gut pain.

I explore the treatment of irritable bowel syndrome in chapter 15, but for now it is a good example of a typical functional disorder, which can affect up to one in five people.

VERO

When I first met Vero, she was in excellent health. Unfortunately, her beloved husband was dying. As I watched them deal with the challenges of a fatal condition, I was struck by her tender and dedicated care. However, things changed dramatically for Vero after his death. She was plunged into a deep grief and, alarmingly, started to collapse. She was brought in to see me by her boss, who was increasingly concerned that his usually excellent and capable worker was being rendered disabled by these periods of unconsciousness. Repeated trips to hospital by ambulance, numerous brain and heart scans, blood tests and monitoring found no abnormality.

Gradually, I got to know more about Vero. Her recent bereavement was not the first difficulty she'd had to cope with. Her childhood was blighted by a 'Cinderella' setting: her biological mother had not been able to raise her and she was sent to her aunt, who resented the obligation to have to care for another child. She had to share a room with her cousin, who abused her. When she tried to tell her aunt, she was rebuffed. As the abuse got worse, Vero would 'black out' (dissociate) during the assaults. Somehow, she got through. An exceptionally bright woman, she managed to get a scholarship and, after university, married quickly and moved as far away from home as possible. All was well, until her husband died. The stress and the grief triggered her previous coping mechanism and she started to black out again.

I have been present during her dramatic collapses. One minute Vero was talking normally but with emotion, the next minute she was slumping to the floor, unrousable. Could they just be faints? This is easy to diagnose because fainting is caused by a fall in blood pressure. I could assert that Vero's pulse, blood pressure and other vital signs remained normal during her periods of unconsciousness. But she did not respond to vigorous efforts to wake her. Her body was totally normal, including her reflexes, but she could not respond. Interestingly, she told me afterwards that she could hear what was being said, even though she was unable to react. This might suggest to you that she was faking it. But this is not the case. Vero had to make strenuous efforts to recover from these blackouts and after several months she ceased having blackouts altogether.[7] (I come back to Vero's story and her recovery through this book.)

Vero's experience is classed as a somatic stress disorder, which is the most severe and disabling form of functional conditions. The history of each person with a somatic stress disorder is unique. Their symptoms cannot be easily categorised and so, often, these patients suffer from a lack of a diagnosis. Without a clear diagnosis, they frequently are shunted from doctor to doctor or make their way through various alternative therapies, with varying levels of relief.

---

[7] In her brilliant book *Functional Somatic Symptoms in Children and Adolescents*, Professor Kasia Kozlowska describes several primitive defensive reflexes that occur in different animals, including the famous 'playing possum', where, under some threat, the animal will assume a stiff or flaccid response to discourage a predator. This reflex may well exist in humans as such responses are well reported in the literature.

The stories of these last three individuals reveal the range of functional conditions, from Min's relatively minor localised symptom to Michael's chronic condition, through to Vero's alarming and incapacitating disorder. All three patients underwent a series of tests, which were normal. Their recovery came not from focusing on the symptom and what it might signify, but on the factors that contributed to their symptoms developing in the first place.

Through the rest of this book, I uncover and explain what these factors are, how they cause these conditions to arise and what can be done to treat them.

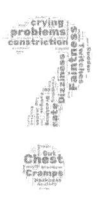

Chapter 3

What causes functional illness?

Your wonderful human body is an incredibly fine-tuned organism of interacting systems that work to maintain everything in your body within healthy parameters: not too cold or overheated, pulse just right, and so on. But what happens when these interacting systems go a bit haywire? Well, do you want the short answer or the long one?

'OK, just give me the bottom line'

If you want the short answer: your functional symptom is a physical stress response. A stress response occurs when your usual state is disrupted by some event – for example, an illness, excessive physical demands, psychological stressors or exhaustion. The body strives to restore order by turning on mechanisms to help you survive the threat. This can produce many different types of symptoms. The symptom can be fleeting, or if the stressful situation is severe or prolonged, your defence mechanisms get turned on and fail to turn off, causing a disruption in the normal way your body responds.

'Alright, what is the whole story?'

Assuming that you are not satisfied with the overly simplistic answer, it is now necessary to introduce you to the complexities of how the brain and the various systems of the body react to each other to cause symptoms.

Before we explore how a functional symptom might arise, it is necessary to understand how your body keeps in balance and good function throughout your life and deals with the various threats or challenges it faces.

How you keep your body in balance

The process by which your body keeps itself in balance is called *homeostasis*. When something disturbs the balance within the body, the systems try to restore the balance by activating the stress response systems – that is, by sensing the change and reacting to restore balance.

Your body can adjust to living in markedly varied environments, from the searing dry heat of the Australian outback to the frozen wastes of the polar regions. Using a wide range of sensors throughout the body, the nervous and hormonal systems respond to maintain balance.

For example, if you are exposed to cold weather, your temperature sensors identify cooling in your skin and so send a message to your brain. This triggers your body stress systems (called your 'defensive mode') which turns on the emergency responses required to keep you warm – for example, you start shivering involuntarily to generate heat, and tiny muscles pull your body hair into goose bumps to keep a layer of warm air near your skin. Several other systems are switched on to deal with the cold stress, and this is how humans have adapted to live all over the world. These are all functional symptoms that are helpful to our wellbeing.

If you are lucky enough to find shelter and warmth soon after being exposed to the cold, your system returns to normal operating mode, which is referred to as the 'maintenance and restorative mode' or simply the 'restorative mode'.

However, if you spend too long in the cold, your coping mechanisms begin to fail. You would run out of the fuel your body needs to generate heat. Your blood would be shunted away from your extremities (that is, your arms and legs), which start to grow very cold. Eventually, your whole body becomes hypothermic. If help doesn't come, your heart eventually would stop.

The two modes

But, as you are still here, you can be grateful that your body has responded pretty well to various stressors throughout your life. For up to 100 years (or even more), your body can stay alive and in working order, more or less. This is due to several highly dynamic systems, which constantly interact with each other and the environment, switching between two modes: the maintenance and restorative mode, and the defensive mode, triggered when a threat or stressor of some kind is identified.

Note that these are the terms preferred by functional doctors for the two modes. The defensive mode may sound like the 'fight, flight or freeze' state and, of course, these responses are included in the defensive mode. But 'fight, flight or freeze' implies the response is always adaptive, helping us to survive our current threats. If you have a functional symptom, however, you will know that the response of the defensive mode is far from helpful. Also, the defensive mode has many more responses than simply creating 'fight, flight or freeze'. Similarly, the maintenance and restorative mode is not simply 'rest and digest' but includes many physiological and psychological responses that are vital for our wellbeing.

The figure overleaf shows a simplified list of the types of symptoms you might experience when in the two modes.

Symptoms experienced when in restorative mode versus defensive mode

YOUR BODY IN RESTORATIVE MODE	YOUR BODY IN DEFENSIVE MODE
Heart rate slow and regular	Heart racing
Breathing calm and even	Breathing work increased
Mouth moist	Mouth dry
Abdomen relaxed	Abdomen tense
Bowels rumbling	Bowels irregular
Bladder under control	Bladder – poor control
Mind calm and alert	Mind agitated/disocciated
Posture relaxed	Posture defensive
Muscles at ease	Muscles tense
Sleep sound	Sleep quality poor
	Body tingling

Your body should switch back and forth between these modes throughout the day.

When you are in good health, deeply relaxed, with not a worry in the world and surrounded by loving and caring people, content with your situation and wanting nothing but to enjoy the moment, you are in your restorative and maintenance mode.

> For good health, you need to spend most of your time in the restorative mode. This is so important but so often overlooked.

Of course, you need to use your defensive mode to keep yourself alert and quick to react when you are confronted with a situation that could threaten you. Sometimes the challenge will be minimal, like running a few steps to get across a road, with very subtle changes in your heartbeat that settle back down very quickly. But what happens to many of us if we need to speak to a large gathering? We may find that we develop many more symptoms that mean we are in the defensive mode. But we still can recover quickly and return to our restorative mode.

However, if you spend too much time in the defensive mode, you can start to develop functional symptoms, due to the activation of one or more of your seven stress response systems. Worse still, severe ongoing stressors or multiple smaller challenges can precipitate a disruption to this nicely balanced system and your defensive mode can *stay activated*. You are not able to return to your restorative mode, even in sleep.

So, instead of maintaining a nice balance between your two modes, where you get to rest and rejuvenate your mind and body in the restorative mode, with the occasional stimulus of the defensive mode to help protect you, you find that you are nearly always in the defensive mode. This does not mean you are psychologically being defensive. It is an *unconscious* state of arousal of any or all of your seven stress response systems.

So, your seven stress response systems are always ready to protect you but can also trigger unwanted symptoms. I cover these seven systems in much more detail in the next chapter. For now, it is important to recognise your body has different systems that can spring into action when there is a real or perceived threat, immediately switching your body from the relaxed state of the maintenance and restorative mode into the defensive mode.[8]

You don't need to know the finer workings of all the systems, but it is important to understand which of your systems have been disrupted so you can focus on what needs to be done to restore them.

---

8   For more information on how your body maintains a balance between the two modes, search online for 'homeostasis and allostasis'.

IS THE CAUSE OF FUNCTIONAL CONDITIONS JUST STRESS?

If stress is defined in its common meaning, then the answer to whether functional conditions are simply caused by stress is no. But learning what can activate your stress systems can make a world of difference. It is better to think of 'stressors' rather than stress.

Stressors are anything that changes the resting mode of your body or mind. A cold environment or physical illness is a stressor, and so is the worry about a serious illness in a loved one. Some of us inherit a highly sensitive nervous system from a parent and can find our bodies reacting where others do not.

Heart rate can vary enormously in some people. While emotional distress can play a role, so can genetics, other illnesses, environmental and social factors, and even personality. This is a good example of how a functional condition can have many causes – be they psychological, physical and even social – and the treatment must be tailored to the correct problem.

Just as our cardiovascular system can be highly reactive, so can our gut. Children who may struggle to express feelings of distress and anxiety can be more likely to complain of nausea or even vomit. This psychosomatic response can settle as they grow up, even if their mental stressors persevere.

To say 'it's just psychosomatic' is implying that we are all born with the same physiology and a small shift in attitude is all that is needed. That is patently not true. There is a huge variation in babies' genetic makeup and, therefore, immune and hormonal responses, long before psychological habits are developed.

And remember Linus (from the introduction). The cause of his pain was never found.

Nature versus nurture

The variety of temperament seen in humans, right from birth, is the same across all mammals. The skittish horse versus the plodder is one example, and dogs can be another. Dogs bred for aggressive mode, which is referred to as the 'maintenance and restorative mode' or simply the 'restorative mode'.

However, if you spend too long in the cold, your coping mechanisms begin to fail. You would run out of the fuel your body needs to generate heat. Your blood would be shunted away from your extremities (that is, your arms and legs), which start to grow very cold. Eventually, your whole body becomes hypothermic. If help doesn't come, your heart eventually would stop.

The two modes

But, as you are still here, you can be grateful that your body has responded pretty well to various stressors throughout your life. For up to 100 years (or even more), your body can stay alive and in working order, more or less. This is due to several highly dynamic systems, which constantly interact with each other and the environment, switching between two modes: the maintenance and restorative mode, and the defensive mode, triggered when a threat or stressor of some kind is identified.

Note that these are the terms preferred by functional doctors for the two modes. The defensive mode may sound like the 'fight, flight or freeze' state and, of course, these responses are included in the defensive mode. But 'fight, flight or freeze' implies the response is always adaptive, helping us to survive our current threats. If you have a functional symptom, however, you will know that the response of the defensive mode is far from helpful. Also, the defensive mode has many more responses than simply creating 'fight, flight or freeze'. Similarly, the maintenance and restorative mode is not simply 'rest and digest' but includes many physiological and psychological responses that are vital for our wellbeing.

The figure overleaf shows a simplified list of the types of symptoms you might experience when in the two modes.

Symptoms experienced when in restorative mode versus defensive mode

YOUR BODY IN RESTORATIVE MODE	YOUR BODY IN DEFENSIVE MODE
Heart rate slow and regular	Heart racing
Breathing calm and even	Breathing work increased
Mouth moist	Mouth dry
Abdomen relaxed	Abdomen tense
Bowels rumbling	Bowels irregular
Bladder under control	Bladder – poor control
Mind calm and alert	Mind agitated/disocciated
Posture relaxed	Posture defensive
Muscles at ease	Muscles tense
Sleep sound	Sleep quality poor
	Body tingling

Your body should switch back and forth between these modes throughout the day.

When you are in good health, deeply relaxed, with not a worry in the world and surrounded by loving and caring people, content with your situation and wanting nothing but to enjoy the moment, you are in your restorative and maintenance mode.

> For good health, you need to spend most of your time in the restorative mode. This is so important but so often overlooked.

Of course, you need to use your defensive mode to keep yourself alert and quick to react when you are confronted with a situation that could threaten you. Sometimes the challenge will be minimal, behaviour versus the cute little furry playthings are evidence that attitude and response to stimuli are not just 'all in the head'. Any animal breeder knows that behavioural tendencies are highly heritable. Only in the last 300 years have we bred dogs as calm as the pug and as potentially aggressive as the American pit bull terrier, which has now been banned or highly regulated in many countries. That doesn't mean that training is not a huge influence. But genetic influence is often under-recognised.

As a beekeeper, I have learnt that the temperament of bees is highly variable and determined by their genetic makeup. Some bees are aggressive with a propensity to sting at the slightest provocation. This is a problem for any beekeeper – and their neighbours. The simple solution is to find another more peace-loving queen. In a short while, all her progeny are also calm.

Humans are no different – that is, genetics plays a big role in how we respond to the world around us. You inherited many traits via your parents' genes. However, just because you may have inherited a tendency for, say, sweaty palms, that doesn't mean there is nothing you can do about it. You cannot change your genes, but you can ensure you get the best advice to manage your vulnerabilities.

Fortunately, for the socially awkward problem of sweaty palms, some pretty good treatments are available. (These options are covered in chapter 15.) But, for the more difficult functional conditions, you and your healthcare team need to develop a better way to provide care. Functional conditions can be complex and multifactorial and deserve careful diagnosis and treatment.

EPIGENETICS: YOU CAN'T CHANGE YOUR GENES BUT CAN YOU PREVENT THEIR EXPRESSION?

While the genes given to you at conception remain unchanged throughout your life, whether your body expresses those genes is dependent on many factors. The tantalising question is this: can you, by altering your environment, both externally and internally, modify the expression of unhelpful genes?

To understand more about this fascinating area of research, we can again look at the bee species. Worker bees and their queen bee have identical genes, but the former are smaller and have a different shape from the queen, who can lay eggs. How does this happen? Current understanding is the impact of royal jelly, the unique substance fed to the larva intended to become a queen. Royal jelly induces the expression of genes that create the body and physiology of a queen.

Studies have shown epigenetic DNA changes in lab rats that were stressed in their infancy, but this is harder to prove in humans, given our complex influences.

So, how is this extraordinary natural phenomenon relevant to you? Is it possible that your early environment caused the expression of certain genes that leave you vulnerable to functional symptoms? The honest answer is that we don't yet know, but it is possible that how you currently live will also affect the expression of your genes, for better or worse.

We certainly know that developing healthy lifestyles have a positive impact on your wellbeing. How much of this is due to epigenetics remains an open question.

Your seven stress response systems

As mentioned, when your body enters defensive mode, one or more of your seven stress response systems are activated. Briefly, the systems and their normal functions are:

1. *Autonomic nervous system:* This controls the bodily functions that are not under your conscious control, such as breathing, heartbeat and digestive processes.
2. *Hormone system:* This sends messages via feedback loops between your brain and other organs using a large number of hormones, each with a different message. This includes your hypothalamic–pituitary–adrenal (HPA) axis,[9] which connects

---

[9] The HPA axis is mediated by neurotransmitters as well as hormones.. A more complete description is found here: https://images.app.goo.gl/H7w8d2rsFbw5EXwt9.

your brain to your adrenal glands and controls reactions to stressors. Many of your bodily functions, such as energy expenditure, emotional regulation, immune activity, gut function, sexual activity and storage of energy, are governed by your HPA. Using both nerves and hormones, the HPA communicates between your brain and body organs and glands.

3. *Immune-inflammatory system:* You need your immune system to help identify and destroy harmful substances or infections. An inflammatory response occurs in your body as part of your defence system protecting against harm from chemicals, irritants, damaged cells or germs; sometimes, however, it is triggered by simply some stressor.

4. *Circadian system:* Your circadian rhythm repeats roughly every 24 hours, coordinating your biological clock and setting your hormone and brain systems to optimise your functioning during night and day.

5. *Skeletomotor system:* When you experience any type of stressor, your skeletomotor system turns on, adopting the muscle tone and posture you need to defend or protect yourself. After the threat has passed your skeletomotor system typically deactivates.

6. *Microbiome–gut–brain system:* This system includes the microbiota (the organisms living in the gut), the gut itself, the communication pathways between the gut and the brain, and relevant regions in the brain (including the brain stress systems).

7. *Brain system:* All the preceding components of your body stress system are coordinated and responded to via the brain system.

> The brain system includes your conscious mind, but up to 95 per cent of the brain system runs automatically in the background.

It's a bit like the computer I am using to type this. The words are the 'conscious' element but most of the computer is functioning without my awareness.

These seven systems operate night and day to keep your body in good condition. But when they get disrupted, problems arise. In the following chapter, I look at how each of these body stress systems can get disrupted and what happens in your body.

THE INVENTION OF STRESS

Did you know that the concept of stress was introduced only in 1956? Hungarian émigré endocrinologist Dr Hans Selye took a term previously used in physics to describe a force upon an object and applied this to human experience. In one regard, it is an unfortunate term, because it has been conflated with another physics term, strain, which is the *effect* of the stress upon the object. However, its use has been universally adopted, and 'stress' (or 'stressor') is now used for any event, whether physical, chemical or psychological, that causes the body to activate your body stress systems. But the situation or mental state that causes a change should be seen as separate from the range of responses you can have.

If, for example, you are suddenly aware of an angry shouting person nearby (the stress or stressor), you can choose from a variety of responses: ignore, move away, laugh it off, attack, soothe, make inquires and so on. The stress is the prompt to action. Your response can be skilful and adaptive or reflexive and aggravating. We often assume that our response to a stressful situation is the only response. So, we might say we are really stressed. But, looking more closely, we can see we might have chosen to respond in a way that was less disruptive to our body stress systems.

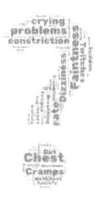

Chapter 4

The seven stress response systems

In the previous chapter, I introduced the two modes your body can switch between – the restorative mode and the defensive mode. Your defensive mode is triggered when your body senses a stressor of some kind, and so activates one of your seven stress systems in response.

In this chapter, I take you on a brief tour of these stress response systems, and how they operate in the two modes. I also introduce you to some of my patients who have experienced unhelpful responses (functional symptoms), generated by the defensive mode.

Autonomic nervous system

When the heart is affected, it reacts on the brain; and the state of the brain again reacts through the pneumo-gastric [vagus] nerve on the heart; so that under any excitement there will be much mutual action and reaction between these, the two most important organs of the body.

Charles Darwin, *The Expression of Emotions in Man and Animals*, 1872

Over 150 years ago, Charles Darwin observed the neurological connection between mind and body. Let's explore some of the ways they talk to each other.

Humans have two separate but interactive nervous systems: the voluntary or somatic nervous system, and the involuntary or autonomic nervous system. The voluntary system is better understood because it is the one consciously controlled: if you want to open or close your hand, you send a message from your brain to your muscles via your somatic nervous system and your hand moves. Immediately after birth, a baby's limbs move in a purposeless, uncontrolled fashion, but over the first year of life she has taught herself to program her brain so that walking, talking and feeding herself is usually achieved. What a triumph!

The autonomic nervous system runs in parallel to your somatic nervous system. It is controlled by parts of the brain that are not immediately under conscious control, and connects to activities such as heart rate, gut function, sweating, hormonal control and breathing, which is fortunate. Imagine having to remember to take every breath. Since your very first breath, the breathing centre in your brain has taken control over the rate and depth of breathing. This exquisitely fine, feedback-controlled system can identify if your oxygen level is too low – say, on a high mountain or after exertion – and, automatically, makes your body breathe more deeply until oxygen levels are restored. Then breathing returns to a base level. Of course, you can override the system and consciously change your breathing – for example, by taking some anticipatory deep breaths before a demanding task.

Your autonomic nervous system is responding second by second to your environment, both internal and external, and activating stress responses as needed. And when the challenge has passed, your system typically switches back to its resting state or restorative mode. But if you have ongoing or overwhelming stressors, especially if they are unpredictable and uncontrollable or even simply recurrent, and you don't get time to deactivate the defensive mode, your autonomic nervous system may remain activated all the time, triggering a permanent defensive mode in your body.

The following figure shows a simplified picture of this autonomic nervous system activation, much of which will likely be familiar to you.

Changes during autonomic nervous system activation

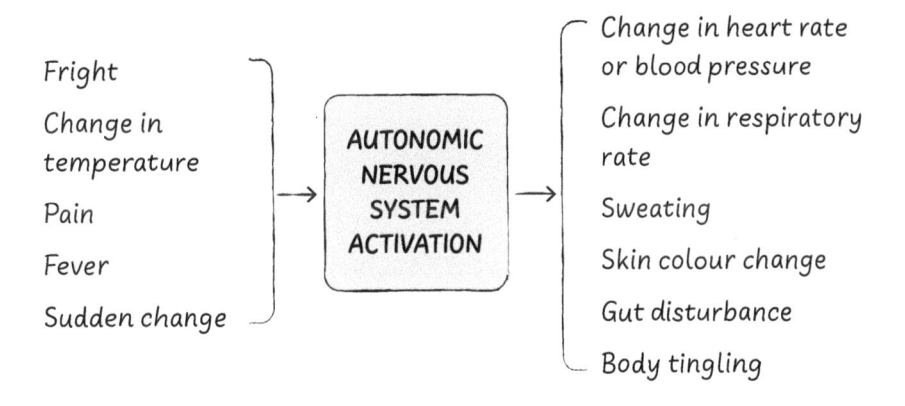

Fright
Change in temperature
Pain
Fever
Sudden change

→ AUTONOMIC NERVOUS SYSTEM ACTIVATION →

Change in heart rate or blood pressure
Change in respiratory rate
Sweating
Skin colour change
Gut disturbance
Body tingling

Your stress response system cannot distinguish between external physical threats and internal, even subconscious, emotional threats. Your body will simply respond with activation of your stress systems.

And the separation between your conscious, somatic nervous system and your automatic autonomic system isn't so clear-cut either. Many actions are carried out by the somatic system without conscious effort. Even walking or talking, which are usually considered to be under voluntary control, are largely done without conscious input. Imagine if you had to plan every movement of your mouth to shape words or every coordination of your leg muscles to walk! The vast majority of human activities are, in fact, conducted by subconscious parts of our brain, with little tweaks from our volitional mind via the voluntary or somatic nervous system.

Because this is the case, you should not be surprised if symptoms sometimes arise out of these involuntary, subconscious parts of your brain.

The autonomic nervous system and functional symptoms

One of the main systems affected by your autonomic nervous system is your cardiovascular system, which is reacting every second of your life to the demands on the body – whether this demand is to increase the flow of blood to muscles doing some hard work or to shunt a good blood supply to the gut to facilitate digestion. The heart and blood vessels that make up the cardiovascular system also react to any emotional stimuli. When we turn 'red with anger' or 'white with fear', this is driven by the autonomic nervous system, which is, in turn, reacting to stimuli from deep parts of the brain where the emotions originate, even if we are not conscious of them.

Blushing is another example. This occurs as a natural response to shame, embarrassment or other emotions. So, when you blush, you have activated your autonomic nervous system via your defensive mode.

The degree to which an individual reacts to a stimulus is determined both by the intensity of the emotion, and by the intensity of the cardiovascular response to even mild emotions. Everyone has felt their heart leap in response to a fright. For most of us, our heart rate will settle back to its normal rate once the fright has passed. But what if our response was to go into prolonged palpitations every time? It's like the sympathetic nervous system – which helps us respond to dangerous or stressful situations – gets turned on to the maximum response for every stimulus.

> Simply calling this response 'psychosomatic' is simplistic and not very helpful.

After the stressor has gone, the body should turn off the stress response, but we know that, in people with functional conditions, the *stress response systems fail to turn off*. The systems continue to be overactive and dominate and disrupt the body's functioning. It's like your defensive mode has switched identities from a highly trained and disciplined police force to a rampaging mob, causing havoc – and no-one is in control. A disciplined police force identifies and acts against those who are a danger to the community (defensive mode), and then settles back into roles such as directing traffic (restorative mode). A mob, on the other hand, can attack anything in their way, and cause chaos and mayhem. Experts still don't fully understand why some people find their systems have gone haywire. But we do know what can help to restore order.

Ethan's story is a good example of how stress can activate the autonomic nervous system and cause unpleasant and alarming symptoms.

> **ETHAN**
>
> Ethan is a lean and mildly anxious man of 53. He normally enjoys a morning walk, but on this occasion, he found himself alarmingly short of breath. He stopped walking, hoping the feeling would pass. Unfortunately, however, Ethan found to his alarm that his feet were going numb. Terrified he was having a stroke, he called 000 and was taken to hospital by ambulance. He had multiple tests, all of which were normal and, because his symptoms had settled, he was sent to his GP for follow-up.
>
> Looking at the bigger picture revealed some further possible reasons for Ethan's symptoms. Ethan was going through a stressful period when a huge and unexpected tax bill arrived. He noticed that he was sighing often and felt a constricting band around his chest. He felt what we call 'air hunger' – the distressing sensation of not being able to get enough air, leading to taking repeated deep breaths. This led to a lowering of the carbon dioxide levels in the body, which is distinctly unpleasant, because it alters the pH (makes the blood less acidic) and causes the nerves in the body to respond abnormally. The deeper breathing only made matters worse.

> This is because hyperventilation, or over-breathing, can lead to a wide array of symptoms, including the following:
> - tightness in the chest
> - 'air hunger', or the feeling like you can't get enough breath
> - very rapid heartbeat
> - sweating
> - tingling or numbness
> - faintness
> - feeling of unreality
> - visual problems
> - rigid muscles, cramps
> - sudden emotional outburst (for example, crying)
> - feeling too hot or too cold.
>
> Ethan came to see me after this distressing experience, and learnt about the phenomenon of hyperventilation. He downloaded an app to train himself in slow breathing and found this revelatory and very helpful. He was encouraged to practise the slow breathing, but also to return if he had ongoing symptoms.

You will have noticed that Ethan's over-breathing occurred spontaneously without any conscious input. His stress response activated his autonomic nervous system and this led automatically to his over-breathing. As highlighted in this example, too much over-breathing (hyperventilation) can lead to widespread and unpleasant symptoms.

The only good thing about hyperventilation is that the body eventually responds with loss of consciousness, and finally the breathing returns to the basic set point and the pH returns to normal, allowing a full recovery. But this is quite a terrifying experience and could be avoided if the condition was better recognised.

Mild forms of hyperventilation syndrome are common and diagnosis of this syndrome can explain a lot of seemingly peculiar symptoms, such as tingling, head fog and 'fullness of the brain'.

Going for a walk 'to clear the head' is a simple strategy – the physical exertion of walking causes the carbon dioxide to return to normal levels and the body and brain recovers. If you are stuck indoors or too overwhelmed to go for a walk, rebreathing into a paper bag will achieve a similar result. The rebreathing of the exhaled carbon dioxide allows the body and brain to restore normal pH and the neuronal disturbance eases.

For more information and tips on slow breathing, see chapter 14.

The hormone system and hypothalamic–pituitary–adrenal axis

All your stress response systems work closely with the vast and complex neural network and hormone system that regulates your organs.

The hormonal system works to power the stress response and mobilise sources of energy for the fight, flight or freeze actions.[10] But, in the process, whenever you are under threat, or simply working too hard, feel upset, lose your cool, get unwell or don't get enough sleep, your stress hormones disrupt the usual functioning of many systems in the body. As a result of your stress response, you shut down your digestion, growth and repair functions, you reduce your sex hormones and, consequently, disrupt your normal sexual function and, if you are a woman, your menstrual cycle.

The figure overleaf highlights the symptoms of a disturbed hormone system.

---

10 Here's a simplified summary of this extraordinarily complex system. The major hormone system involved in stress responses is the sympathetic–adrenal–medullary (SAM) axis, which is fired to release stress hormones such as adrenaline within seconds from the adrenal medulla. Within minutes of the perceived threat, the hypothalamus–pituitary–adrenal (HPA) axis is triggered as well and the adrenal glands start to pump out steroids. A further stimulus arrives at the adrenal gland, via the pituitary which releases another hormone, CRF (corticotropin-releasing factor). CRF, in turn, signals the secretion of adrenocorticotropin hormone (ACTH) also from the pituitary. ACTH also travels to the adrenal gland where it stimulates the production of more glucocorticoids such as cortisol.

Symptoms caused by a disturbed hormone system

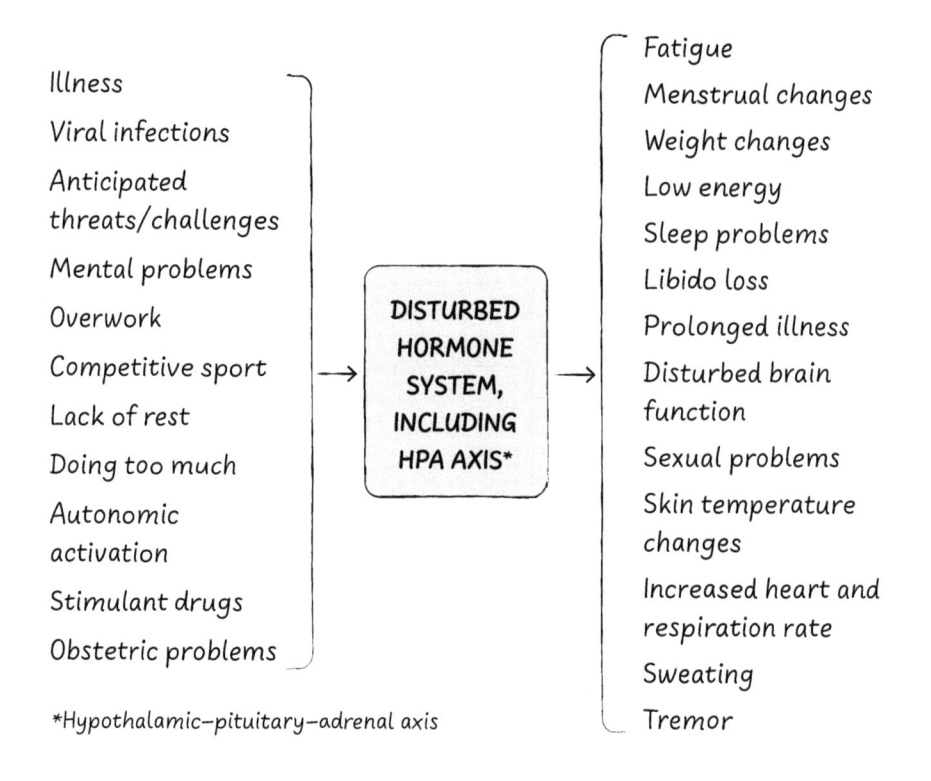

Inputs (stressors):
- Illness
- Viral infections
- Anticipated threats/challenges
- Mental problems
- Overwork
- Competitive sport
- Lack of rest
- Doing too much
- Autonomic activation
- Stimulant drugs
- Obstetric problems

→ **DISTURBED HORMONE SYSTEM, INCLUDING HPA AXIS*** →

Symptoms:
- Fatigue
- Menstrual changes
- Weight changes
- Low energy
- Sleep problems
- Libido loss
- Prolonged illness
- Disturbed brain function
- Sexual problems
- Skin temperature changes
- Increased heart and respiration rate
- Sweating
- Tremor

*Hypothalamic–pituitary–adrenal axis

The brain is the source of the immediate and ongoing release of stress hormones that, in turn, disrupt the normal functioning of the body. Your whole body switches from restorative mode to defensive mode. And your stress hormones appear to have an impact on the prefrontal cortex, which is the part of your brain critical for much of the more demanding, executive mental functioning. This means the release of stress hormones may reduce your cognitive skills and coping strategies. Have you ever felt that you can't think straight? This may be due to your stress hormones.

> Is there any wonder that stressors can have such a profound effect on the healthy functioning of mind and body?

Not only does stress affect hormone levels, but the normal hormone changes in the body also have an impact on symptoms. Women with functional conditions will often notice a cyclical variation in their symptoms in tune with their menstrual cycle. Menopause and the sudden change in sex hormone levels can lead to new symptoms, such as sleep disturbance and mood changes. These and other symptoms can place an extra strain on women dealing with functional conditions.

The critical influence of your hypothalamus

The hypothalamus is where your conscious and subconscious perceptions of your environment interact with the rest of the brain and your body. Imagine you have just seen a large spider in your bedroom and your fear of spiders has triggered a strong defensive mode response. You need to notify the rest of your body of the threat. You automatically send a message to your hypothalamus, which sends a cascade of neurotransmitters and stress hormones down to the pituitary, a tiny but vital gland on the bottom of your brain. In turn, it sends more stress hormones to your adrenal glands on top of your kidneys, which sets in train a release of yet more stress hormones such as adrenaline and cortisol, and you feel your heart start racing and your muscles tense. You have activated your hypothalamic–pituitary–adrenal (HPA) axis.

So the hypothalamus is the control centre that governs the release of hormones from the pituitary gland at the base of the brain. These hormones also regulate the reproductive system and control the release of the sex hormones. During a stressful time, the hypothalamus can shut down the flow of hormones and disrupt hormone levels necessary for fertility. Even relatively innocuous stressors, such as exams or holidays, can cause hormone changes that lead to menstrual periods becoming intermittent or even non-existent.

Any man who has ever found himself suddenly unable to perform in his usual sexual capacity may be experiencing a functional disruption to his erectile potency through his stress hormones. If your body believes it is fighting for your life, it is not going to allow any diversion of energy to secondary functions such as sex. In this situation, problems with getting an erection may be a functional symptom.

The HPA axis is an amazing survival system, but it can be disrupted. Kirralee's story is a dramatic version of an over-activated HPA system.

KIRRALEE

When I first met 30 year old Kirralee, it was obvious that she was scared out of her wits. For the last several nights, she had been waking with her heart feeling like it was leaping out of her chest. She had been to the hospital repeatedly, each time thinking she was going to die.

She would spend the wee hours in hospital, having test after test, only to be sent home in the morning, exhausted but with her heart back to normal speed. This would repeat night after night.

Kirralee was having panic attacks, which can cause truly terrifying symptoms (see the following section). The only good thing about a panic attack is that it expends its energy rapidly and the body usually recovers its normal condition within a few hours.

For a long time, Kirralee struggled to see the connection between her internal mental milieu and the palpitations. She was convinced that something was catastrophically wrong with her heart and she insisted on numerous referrals to cardiologists. These tests ruled out physical diseases, however, and all Kirralee's symptoms pointed to the likelihood of an activated HPA axis.

The important thing to note here is that the whole process was proceeding without Kirralee being aware of it. She was not aware of the impact of her past traumas – she was living far away from all that, working full-time and enjoying her relationship, and she believed that she had left it far behind.

She was not aware of the stressors causing her to develop her symptoms until too late – she was focused on her work and family. She was not aware that the mortal fear that drove her to the hospital and the heart specialists was the very thing she needed to master if she was to feel better.

During her traumatic childhood, Kirralee had learnt to rely on herself and remain hypervigilant to avoid danger. She was not aware that this very inner tension and heightened awareness, rather than being protective now, was causing muscle spasms, chest pain, palpitations and terror. So, she ended up in the emergency room thinking she was having a heart attack, again. And her very fear of dying was actually making her sicker by further triggering her HPA response.

I outline what Kirralee did to overcome her panic attacks and this heightened HPA response in chapter 5.

The HPA axis and functional symptoms

If you have ever had a panic attack, you would know that the unpleasant symptoms can arise as if out of nowhere. A panic attack is a horrible and scary experience. According to the Victorian Government's Better Health Channel, symptoms of a panic attack can include the following:

- heightened vigilance for danger and physical symptoms
- anxious and irrational thinking
- a strong feeling of dread, danger or foreboding
- fear of going mad, losing control, or dying
- feeling lightheaded and dizzy
- tingling and chills, particularly in the arms and hands
- trembling or shaking, sweating
- hot flushes
- accelerated heart rate
- a feeling of constriction in the chest
- breathing difficulties, including shortness of breath
- nausea or abdominal distress

- tense muscles
- dry mouth
- feelings of unreality and detachment from the environment.

You'll notice symptoms in common here with hyperventilation, because over-breathing is part of panic.

It is totally understandable that many people end up in the emergency department of their nearest hospital. It is important to be sure it is 'only' a panic attack, because serious health conditions, such as a heart attack, can present in a similar way. But emergency services may not give the diagnosis of panic attack. The reason for this is that it is not the job of the hospital to make diagnoses, but to rule out serious conditions. This is aided by the eventual return to normal that most panic attack sufferers experience.

But let us look more closely at the cause of these attacks. For many people, they seem to arise out of the blue – for example, standing in a queue in the supermarket or sitting at home. There is no obvious threat at the time. This unpredictability makes them even more alarming, so it feels like it must be a heart attack or some similar life-threatening event.

Only in retrospect can some people become aware that they are contending with some form of stressor or existential threat. (And, sometimes, they never find a cause.) At the time, they may be fixed on solving the problem, and getting rid of the symptoms. But in doing so they can get caught in a vicious cycle – they may be unaware of the common stressors (such as lack of sleep or too much work) and how potently they can activate emergency responses in the body. Additionally, the more they focus on their panic symptoms, the worse they become. This internal stress on the HPA causes a flood of chemicals, such as adrenaline, to surge throughout the body, which responds by turning on the fight, flight or freeze emergency response. Once the adrenaline is pumping, little can be done until the episode has passed, except remember that it will pass without any lasting effects.

> Remember – when it comes to chest pain, especially if it persists for minutes, prompt action may save your life. It is not a good time to wonder if an unconscious process is causing you to develop chest pain.
> Just call an ambulance.

Usually harmless symptoms, but horrible to endure

Functional symptoms are real symptoms, but all the usual tests after a panic attack, for example, shows a totally normal healthy body. No signs suggest whether another attack is likely.

Again, it is important to remember here that the tests performed in hospitals are designed solely to identify physical, not functional, conditions. If Kirralee (from the previous example) was tested for body stress responses, she would have been off the chart! So, when doctors tell you all your tests are normal, this needs to be heard as they have not found a physical diagnosis that could do actual harm to your body. (If a test existed to measure activation of the HPA system, on the other hand, there would be another answer.)

And yet more attacks can occur. While there is no way to predict when, you can overcome these symptoms and gain mastery over your body's responses. I provide more detail on how in part III of this book. For now, an important point to remember is that you don't need to understand the exact mechanism by which these symptoms arise. That twang of pain in the abdomen could be from the bowel or the abdominal muscles or the ureter, but if it goes away quickly, you don't need to worry.

Unfortunately, worry is a common feature of functional conditions. We can be so focused on the task at hand that we fail to recognise how the stress of the task is affecting our functioning. This is particularly so for high-functioning, high-achieving individuals who don't allow themselves to acknowledge their own levels of stress. Or, even when they do know they are tired or overdoing it, they force themselves to push on. They stretch themselves until something snaps.

A common theme in functional conditions is that unconscious and reflexive processes are at play.

Broken heart syndrome

Occasionally, the HPA system can be activated to such an extreme that true harm can occur. A very serious functional condition is takotsubo cardiomyopathy or 'broken heart syndrome'. In this condition, a surge of extreme emotion causes the HPA system to put a strain on your heart's main blood-pumping chamber (the left ventricle), which distorts into a shape similar to an octopus trap called 'takotsubo' by Japanese fishermen. This strain and distortion weakens the heart muscle and means it doesn't pump blood as well as it should. It is debatable if this should be called a functional condition, given the very real physical changes in the heart, except that, seconds before the emotional strain, the heart was completely normal.

POTS

POTS, or postural orthostatic tachycardia syndrome, is another condition caused by an over-activated HPA system. You may have had a taste of what this condition feels like when you first got up after a bout of illness and your heart raced and you felt unsteady. People with POTS experience a racing heart whenever they stand, and this can be associated with a lot of disabling symptoms such as light-headedness, poor concentration, fatigue and other problems. These symptoms can mean they are unable to work or study. The quality of life in POTS patients is comparable to patients on dialysis for kidney failure.

Tests show a perfectly normal heart and normal blood results, but the culprit is an over-activated HPA system and disruption to the autonomic nervous system.

Dr Kozlowska and her team at the Westmead Hospital Mind-Body Program have developed a fascinating approach to working with young people with POTS, focusing on redressing the disturbance of the autonomic nervous system – for more information on this, see chapter 14.

Immune-inflammatory system

Your immune system is what helps your body recognise foreign elements, such as bacteria and viruses, and destroy them. It does this by being able to recognise 'self' and 'non-self' – anything 'non-self' needs to be destroyed. If you suffer from allergies, your immune system is also reacting to harmless elements – for example, dust – in an unhelpful way. In this case, the immune system will overreact to the innocuous dust, causing a cascade of symptoms. Across the human population, a vast variety of responses can be identified to these stimuli. In the recent COVID epidemic, for example, some people had no infection, some tested positive for the infection but showed no signs (asymptomatic infection), while those showing signs of infection suffered anything from a mild sniffle to an overwhelming and even fatal infection. Then, some of those infected have gone on to develop prolonged illness following their COVID infection. So, humans have a vast variety of immune responses and this applies to every infection.

We also have highly variable immune responses to stimuli other than infections, such as foods, chemicals, ultraviolet rays, drugs, emotions and sleep deprivation, which may be the reason some people suffer symptoms in situations where others will not.

But did you know that if your defensive mode is activated (that is, your body has switched from restorative mode), changes in your immune-inflammatory system might also be triggered, leading to inflammation, rashes, swelling and pain? This system can be activated independently from your psychological experience – that is, your defensive mode preferentially activates your immune-inflammatory system, rather than your brain system.

The following figure shows possible symptoms caused by a disruption to the immune-inflammatory system.

Possible symptoms caused by a disruption to the immune-inflammatory system

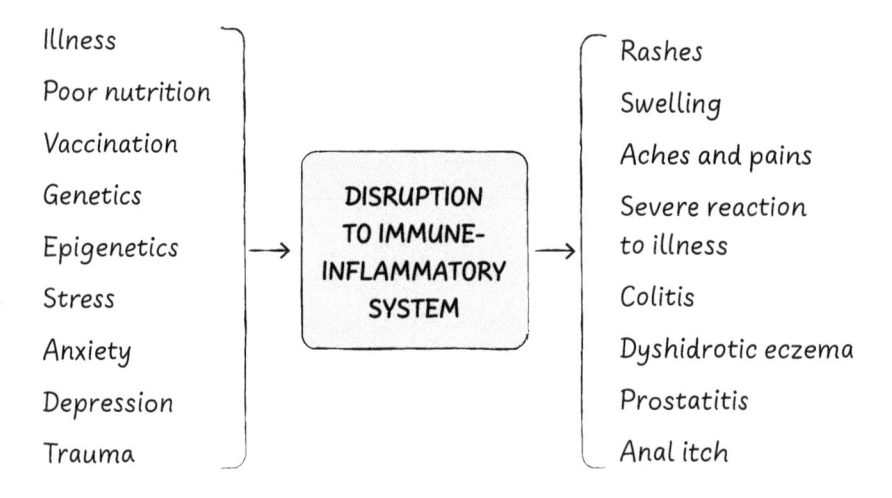

Inputs		Outputs
Illness		Rashes
Poor nutrition		Swelling
Vaccination		Aches and pains
Genetics	DISRUPTION TO IMMUNE-INFLAMMATORY SYSTEM	Severe reaction to illness
Epigenetics		
Stress		Colitis
Anxiety		Dyshidrotic eczema
Depression		Prostatitis
Trauma		Anal itch

What has the immune system to do with functional conditions? Experts don't have the full answer, but some fascinating new findings are helping to unlock the mysteries around unexplained symptoms such as inflammation and pain.

The immune system is intricately connected to the brain in many ways. Every neurone has immune cells nearby to protect it and the blood flowing through all parts of the brain carry immune cells and antibodies and all the other elements that make up the immune system.

If you get eczema or hives, you likely know this is an immune reaction occurring in the skin. This can be caused by allergies but also simply stress. Perhaps you also have unusual brain reactions with stress. Could this be immune-mediated? Some interesting research findings are emerging in this area, however, we are far from a clear understanding about these mechanisms.

The various pathways by which these effects are mediated are extremely complex and perpetually interact with other elements in the body. There are negative feedback loops, cascading accelerations of inflammatory responses, immediate responses and delayed responses. The responses also change if they continue for longer than usual. For example, cortisol is released as a response to acute stress, but prolonged stress leads to a dampened cortisol response, which may explain that morning struggle to wake up and get going.

Understanding the role of the immune system in functional conditions may help future treatments. However, having studied the immune system for over 40 years, I feel that trying to fix it by adjusting one element is like pulling a thread in a tightly knotted ball of wool. It doesn't help.

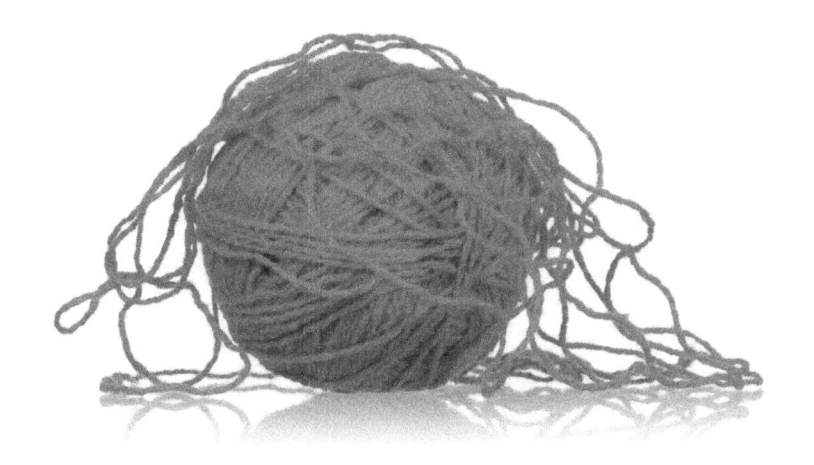

Recent research has revealed that if you have activated your stress response system, major changes occur in your immune-inflammatory system. The full complexity behind this is beyond the scope of this book, but an important aspect to focus on is one of the white cells, called macrophages (Greek for 'big eaters'). These normally travel around your body and eat any debris, dead cells or foreign particles, and they secrete anti-inflammatory molecules to turn off inflammation.

But when your body turns on its defensive mode, the macrophages can 'go rogue' (see the following figure[11]) and start to excrete

---
11 Images derived from Dr Kozlowska's work.

inflammatory molecules and play a role in increasing your pain and swelling. This means some of your aches and pains may be caused by your own immune system stuck in defensive mode.

Restorative mode macrophage   *Defensive mode macrophage*

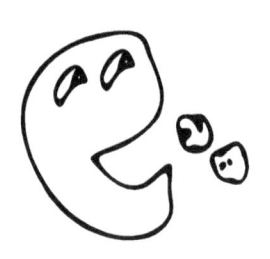

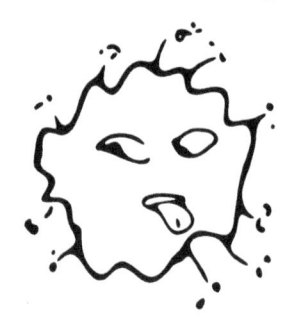

Recent research has also highlighted the importance of exercise and physical activity in returning your body to its healthy restorative mode.[12] This activity helps the macrophages to return to their normal job and start excreting anti-inflammatory molecules again, which will reduce your pain. So, this is one reason you may find that prolonged inactivity leaves you feeling stiff and sore but a return to even gentle exercise can help relieve this pain. The process is like turning on your internal source of anti-inflammatory treatment.

Your doctor may have encouraged you to be active daily. But do you struggle to commit to this because of the effort required? Again, understanding the complex science behind the benefits of exercise is not necessary. However, it may help to know that exercise is not simply good for you, but it will make you feel better. (See chapter 14 for more on the benefits of exercise and how to increase daily physical activity skillfully and safely.)

Your immune-inflammatory system can also play a critical role in modulating your pain in other ways. From receptors in the skin, to tiny chemical signals to the pain nerve fibres and spinal cord

---

12 In her brilliant book *Functional Somatic Symptoms in Children and Adolescents*, Professor Kasia Kozlowska describes several primitive defensive reflexes that occur in different animals.

right up to parts of your brain where pain is actually experienced, all these elements interact with every other system, causing pain to arise. For example, stress-induced activation of the skeletomotor system can lead to pain in tense and taut muscles, which can be a source of serious pain. And yet the usual tests used to identify physical sources of pain will be normal.

In chapter 5, I examine the pain system in more detail.

> **PSYCHONEUROENDOIMMUNOLOGY**
>
> Some fascinating discoveries have emerged in the field of psychoneuroendoimmunology (or PNEI for short – yes, it's a mouthful). This area of study incorporates findings from research into the effects of stressors on the nervous system, the hormone system and the immune system, and looks at how they all interact to create changes in the body.
>
> One of the many powers of the human brain is its capacity for prescience: it can predict a threat and mount a defence in readiness of attack. But the brain will respond to real or imagined threats in the same way – and then, given the state of readiness, the stress response plays out in the immune-inflammatory system as low level inflammation. Your doctor's usual tests for inflammation are negative, but subtle changes can be identified.
>
> By communication with other stress response systems in patients with chronic pain, the immune-inflammatory system keeps the pain system activated and signalling pain.
>
> Fatigue systems are also possibly activated, but the research here is still needed.

Circadian rhythm

Your sleep/wake cycle, called your circadian rhythm, is vital for allowing your body to repair and rejuvenate itself. This cycle also works closely with your hormone system and any disruptions can impair your health. If you have ever done shift work or had jet lag, you would know about this. Your gut hormones are also affected by your circadian rhythm and when it is disrupted, you may develop nausea, indigestion, constipation, diarrhoea and defecation at unusual times.

The disruption to your sleep patterns is not often seen as the cause for ongoing poor health, so the worry about a decline in your health can aggravate the vicious cycle.

> Good-quality sleep is essential to create the ultimate restorative and maintenance mode. This is when your body really gets a chance to repair, rejuvenate and restore itself each night.

And, yes, you need around eight hours of quality sleep to achieve this. If you are waking unrefreshed, stiff and sore, you may not be achieving an adequately restorative state.

The following figure shows possible symptoms caused by a disruption to your circadian rhythm.

Shift workers experience a chronic stress upon their bodies, with frequent disruptions to their systems that can lead to activation of the immune-inflammatory system and dysregulation of the autonomic nervous system. (See earlier in this chapter for more on these systems.)

Sleep deprivation and the circadian rhythm

Sleep deprivation is such a common phenomenon now, whether it is due to longer commute times or maybe just the use of devices at bedtime. These factors are so common that people of all ages often fail to realise how harmful they are for their general wellbeing.

Possible symptoms caused by a disruption to the circadian rhythm

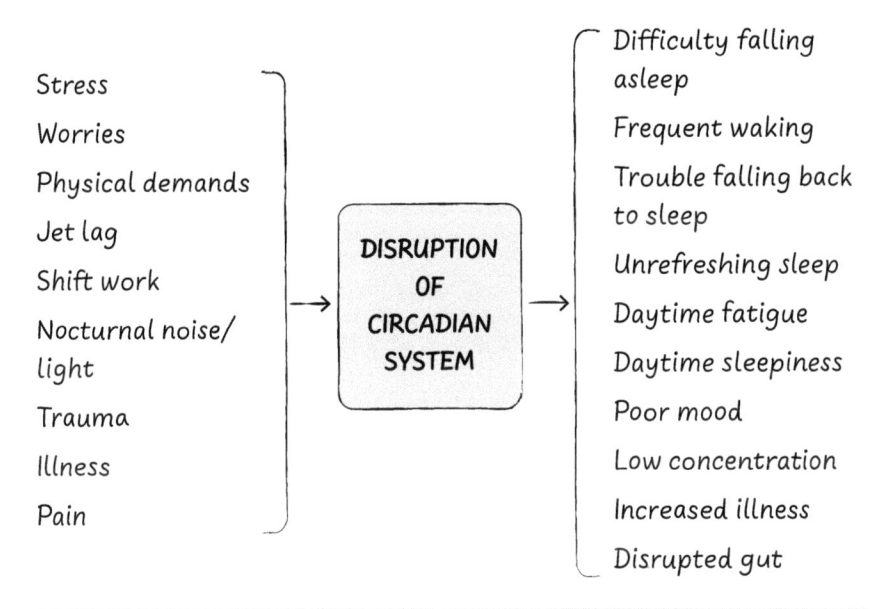

Stress, Worries, Physical demands, Jet lag, Shift work, Nocturnal noise/light, Trauma, Illness, Pain → **DISRUPTION OF CIRCADIAN SYSTEM** → Difficulty falling asleep, Frequent waking, Trouble falling back to sleep, Unrefreshing sleep, Daytime fatigue, Daytime sleepiness, Poor mood, Low concentration, Increased illness, Disrupted gut

LACK OF SLEEP IMPAIRS PERFORMANCE

Let's say that a person who needs eight hours of sleep per night only gets six. According to the Victorian Government's Better Health Channel, this two-hour sleep loss can have a major impact including:

- reduced alertness
- shortened attention span
- slower than normal reaction time
- poorer judgement
- reduced awareness of the environment and situation
- reduced decision-making skills
- poorer memory
- reduced concentration
- increased likelihood of mentally 'stalling' or fixating on one thought
- increased likelihood of moodiness and bad temper
- reduced work efficiency
- loss of motivation
- errors of omission – making a mistake by forgetting to do something

- errors of commission – making a mistake by doing something, but choosing the wrong option
- microsleeping – brief periods of involuntary sleeping that range from a few seconds to a few minutes in duration.

When patients notice such a list of symptoms developing, they commonly request a brain scan to check for more serious problems. They do not often appreciate the advice that they should get more sleep as a first step. The low-level functioning during their day often leads to inefficient and therefore prolonged working hours, adding to the vicious cycle.

Again, the circadian rhythm regulates your body's rest and repair. When your body is in restorative mode, your circadian rhythm will help to optimise all your other systems to restore good health. It is so important to your recovery that I cover functional conditions relating to sleep disorders and fatigue in depth in chapter 6.

Skeletomotor system

Your skeletomotor system is what it says on the label: your muscles, tendons and bones work in a coordinated fashion to get your body to do things. When you are in restorative mode, your skeletomotor system maintains your body movements in a relaxed state and your posture is upright but relaxed. Look at a baby sitting on the floor with a straight spine but happily relaxed limbs and movement.

But if you activate your defensive mode, your brain system instructs your skeletomotor system to protect the body, and especially the head, by hunching the shoulders, ducking your head lower, and tensing your muscles ready for fight, flight or freeze. This ancient survival instinct is playing out in the modern workplace, with the resultant poor posture, headaches and muscle tension being commonplace.[13]

---

13 Aching behind the eyes often prompts an eye check, but it is sometimes due to referred pain from tight neck muscles.

But a severe aggravation of your defensive mode can cause not only tension, but also weakness or even paralysis. These alarming symptoms can lead to a vicious cycle of further brain system activation and a highly aroused stress response. None of these activation pathways utilise the conscious parts of the brain and, therefore, can be difficult to resolve.

The following figure shows possible symptoms caused by an over-activated skeletomotor system.

Possible symptoms caused by an activated skeletomotor system

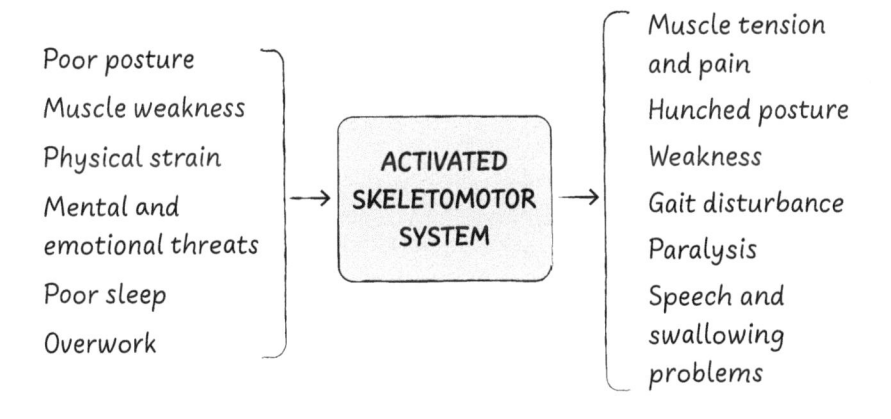

Inputs to ACTIVATED SKELETOMOTOR SYSTEM:
- Poor posture
- Muscle weakness
- Physical strain
- Mental and emotional threats
- Poor sleep
- Overwork

Outputs from ACTIVATED SKELETOMOTOR SYSTEM:
- Muscle tension and pain
- Hunched posture
- Weakness
- Gait disturbance
- Paralysis
- Speech and swallowing problems

ROMANA'S GAIT DISTURBANCE

Romana was brought to see me by his sister, who had been caring for him since he underwent a successful back operation two months earlier. Romana had done well with his inpatient rehabilitation and achieved normal walking and mobilisation. But as he left the hospital building, Romana found his gait 'went weird' and he found himself lurching forward and back. It was frightening and embarrassing in equal measure. In my surgery, I was able to briefly distract him and saw his gait return to normal but as soon as he noticed this, the gait disturbance returned. It was obvious that this was a functional disturbance, but Romana insisted he see one neurologist after another. Disappointed that they couldn't help him and rejecting the idea that his inability to walk could be functional, Romana took months to regain his normal gait.

The real issue that I was not able to address with Romana was the reasons his defensive mode was violently activated as he left the hospital. He was understandably fixated on his gait problem and convinced it was something to do with the surgery. He never accepted that he had not suffered neurological injury, but he eventually found a therapist who was able to help him with restoring his normal gait.

Overactivity or underactivity in the skeletomotor system can disrupt the balance of your systems. As mentioned earlier in this chapter, inactivity can aggravate the inflammatory system and cause pain. If you have pain, you might imagine that you should not be active or use the painful area. And this can be correct for some injuries – say, a sprained ankle. But once the pain has been found to be functional, judicious movement is an important, indeed essential, part of recovery.

And overactivity, such as sudden unaccustomed exercise or extreme physical exertion, can also lead to a massive stress upon all your body stress systems and lead to multiple and serious functional illnesses.

As an example of this, competitive sports can set unrealistic demands upon the body and those who believe that they should relentlessly push way beyond the pain barrier are choosing to ignore their body's warnings.

Your skeletomotor system works hand in hand with your autonomic nervous system, so when you have a stress response due to illness, fear or injury, the autonomic system drives your respiratory muscles to work harder and you may develop hyperventilation (as discussed earlier in this chapter). Similarly, activation of the skeletomotor system during a stress response can lead to abnormal muscle function, called dystonia, which can manifest as voice disturbance, disturbed posture, swallowing difficulties, weakness, or cramp or disturbance of gait, like Romana's.

The microbiota–gut–brain system

Consider the following expressions:

- 'I felt sick at the thought of it.'
- 'Her stomach heaved when she saw the sight.'
- 'It was gut-wrenching.'
- 'My stomach was full of butterflies.'
- 'His mouth went dry when he realised what he'd done.'
- 'I nearly s**t myself.'

All these expressions are examples of obvious functional symptoms. They reveal some of the very visceral ways our minds and our guts interact, but much subtler processes can arise. A sudden change in your situation can show you the obvious connection between your mind and your gut, but the slow burn of persistent low-grade, ordinary, run-of-the-mill stressors can be harder to identify, making it less obvious that your gut symptoms may be related to your usual state of mind.

A more recent area of research has been looking at the effect of changes in the gut bacteria or microbiota on the workings of the brain. Studies show that a healthy diet supports of wide range of gut bacteria or 'flora', which protect and nourish the lining of the gut. Disturbances to the lining, due to a poor diet or certain medication, may cause your functional gut symptoms. The latest research is also focusing on the DNA of this huge number of organisms that live inside us, and the influence of this DNA, or 'microbiome', and its interaction with the brain system.

This could mean, if you have a functional gut disorder, the deregulation of your microbiota–gut–brain system may be the reason. Your gut has a massive nervous system – your brain has only twice as many neurons! So it is understandable that a lot of communication occurs between your gut and your brain, via numerous pathways, including the autonomic nervous system, the pain pathways, hormonal circulation and the result of the microbiota.

> Your gut contains the outside world and is itself the barrier between the world and you. This barrier can be disrupted and this in turn can lead to your immune-inflammatory system becoming involved.

So a healthy and diverse gut microbiota not only helps to ensure good nutrition but also may send messages to the brain via the HPA axis to support its normal function.

You can begin to see how your diet and the health of your gut could affect how your brain functions. The exact mechanism of how nutrition, gut health and your environment all affect your stress systems is being studied with more discoveries being made. For example, by maintaining a healthy quantity of good bacteria, such as lactobacilli (found in yogurt and fermented vegetables), you can help to protect yourself from unhealthy bacterial overgrowth, gut inflammation and functional gut symptoms.

The following figure shows possible symptoms caused by a disrupted microbiota–gut–brain system.

Possible symptoms caused by a disrupted microbiota–gut–brain system

Poor diet
Drugs and alcohol
Gut irritants
Stress
Inactivity
Disrupted sleep
Hormonal changes

→ DISRUPTED MICROBIOTA–GUT–BRAIN SYSTEM →

Abdominal pain and bloating
Nausea
Bowel disturbance
Wind
Brain fog
Malaise
Poor appetite

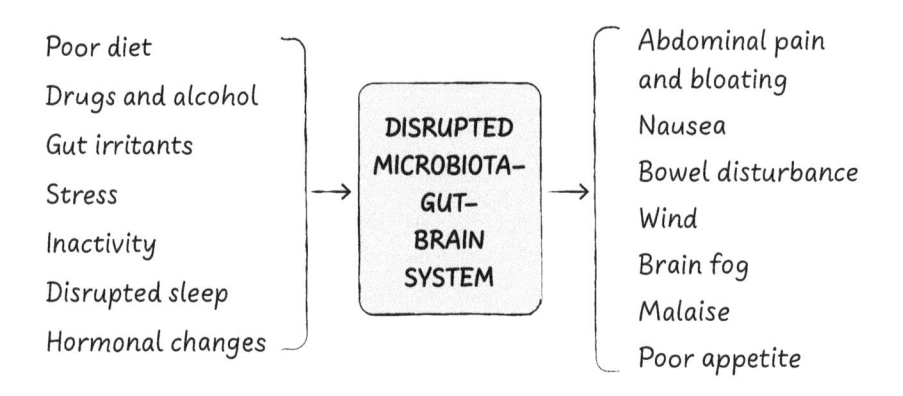

The brain stress system

Of course, your extraordinary brain, the most complex system in the universe, is dealing with all the six systems discussed so far in this chapter. When talking about your brain system, I am mainly referring to the automatic, reflexive parts of your brain, not your conscious, thinking mind. The brain system is the conductor of the orchestra. It hears what every other system is playing and modulates all the systems to respond. When your brain system is in restorative mode, all the other systems are quietly playing in the background and your body is in its optimal state.

Picture yourself relaxing on a sunny day, enjoying a picnic. All your systems are in happy accord. Now imagine what happens when you sit on an ant nest: the ant bites send a pain signal rapidly to your brain system, which responds by reflexively activating your skeleto-motor system to jump off the nest before you even consciously know what has happened. Your immune-inflammatory system immediately gets to work to neutralise the ant bite poison, creating the redness, swelling and pain. The pain site tells your brain system where the bites are and helps you to finally consciously check if any more ants are on you and deal with them.

Meanwhile, your brain system has also activated your HPA system to release more stress hormones to focus your body and mind on the problem and allocate resources to deal with it. If the ant bites are severe, your circadian system will be disrupted that evening and there will be further stress responses. As you can see, nearly every system is activated, all governed by your brain system.

Now, imagine yourself dealing with a very stressful problem in your home. Your brain system is again automatically activated into defensive mode, which results in all your other systems being likewise activated. Most of these responses are automatic and innate. You do not consciously activate them. Your conscious mind is focused on the problem perhaps, but your body is copping the effects of an activated defensive mode. If the stressful problem persists or is severe, your defensive mode stays activated, and functional symptoms are likely to develop.

You don't even need to be facing an overt problem for this to occur. If you have an anxiety or depressive disorder, a similar response of brain system activation can occur, without any external problem being consciously apparent.

Many books can help deal with mental health issues, and I recommend anyone with such issues get professional help. My focus in this book is functional symptoms, which are a common part of mental health problems. The best remedy for these functional symptoms is to deal with the mental condition that may have caused the activation of your defensive mode.

Mental habits that can activate the defensive mode include the following:

- hypervigilance
- negative thinking
- catastrophising
- ruminations
- anxiety
- nocebo effect (see chapter 7).

These mental habits can activate stress responses in your brain stress system and this can lead to the start or maintenance of functional symptoms, as shown in the following figure.

Unlike the ant bite, a mentally stressful situation will also activate your microbiome–gut–brain system, and symptoms such as nausea, gut churning or bowel disturbance can arise. This is particularly so for children, who often get an upset stomach during stress. They may not be able to talk about the stressors so we need to look for clues: if the upset tummy only occurs on Monday morning, for example, we would be expecting some problem at school that is playing out unwittingly through the child's defensive mode.

Possible symptoms caused by an activated brain stress system

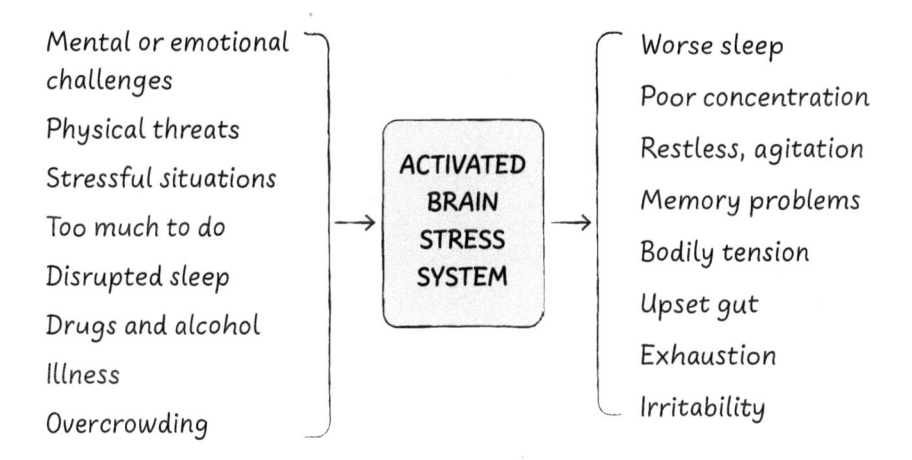

Mental or emotional challenges
Physical threats
Stressful situations
Too much to do
Disrupted sleep
Drugs and alcohol
Illness
Overcrowding

→ **ACTIVATED BRAIN STRESS SYSTEM** →

Worse sleep
Poor concentration
Restless, agitation
Memory problems
Bodily tension
Upset gut
Exhaustion
Irritability

Dissociation – you can run but you can't hide

Some people deal with unwanted memories, feelings or thoughts by putting them out of their conscious mind. This is called 'dissociation', which can be a very helpful coping mechanism in the middle of a problem. But it can also activate your automatic (unconscious) brain stress system, which leads to an increase in your physical stress levels and functional symptoms nevertheless.

Innate defence responses – how we evolved to respond when all else fails

Remember Vero and her collapses from chapter 2? Her brain system was so overwhelmed by her traumas that it would shut down her consciousness and her skeletomotor system entirely. Dr Kasia Kozlowska (working with her team at the Westmead Hospital Mind-Body Program) has documented the different types of innate stress responses we have to threats – fight or flight for example, is when we *actively* respond, while freeze is when fight or flight is put on hold. However, when the threat is overwhelming, two other responses can occur: 'tonic immobility' and 'collapsed immobility' – two types of paralysis.

Tonic immobility is when the body automatically adopts a rigid, frozen posture. This was seen in large numbers of men suffering what was called at the time 'shell shock', when the horrendous conditions on the World War I battlefields overwhelmed the brain system.

Collapsed immobility is when the body appears dead. Vero's involuntary responses to her experience of severe stressors were collapsed immobility. This is an innate response that we all possess and may have experienced briefly – when our legs have given way, for example, in response to a shock. Vero's collapsed immobility could last up to an hour or two, leading to hasty investigations by emergency department doctors worried about brain haemorrhages and other causes of sudden loss of consciousness.

All these responses resolve over time, but can recur – as they did with Vero, who underwent over a dozen CT scans of her brain before the depth of her childhood traumas was revealed, and she received appropriate therapy to enable her to move on.

The bad news and the good news

The bad news is if you have triggered a stress response in one system, it is likely to affect all the other closely interactive systems. So, if you have a stressful night with disrupted sleep, the following day you may have mental dullness, aches or upset digestion or fatigue. Bad.

The good news is that if you focus on improving at least one of your systems, you can bring benefit to all the others. For example, if you focus on calming the mind, you may improve your circadian rhythm, have a more relaxed skeletomotor system and so on.

Many of us are fortunate to be able to return to restorative mode without any effort. But if you have developed a symptom, functional or otherwise, that is not settling, a good place to start is to try to optimise the following health basics:

- ensure adequate hours of deep, restorative sleep
- undertake regular physical activity that is not going to lead to exhaustion that night or the next day

- follow a balanced diet
- remove toxins and disruptors such as alcohol, smoking, recreational drugs and excess caffeine
- begin to notice if your mental habits (*how* you think) are helpful or not when it comes to your response to situations.

I provide much more detail on how to enter the restorative state in part III. For now, this checklist is a good starting point. If you follow these basics, the body and mind have a good chance of operating normally and repairing any minor problems that arise. Nothing is new in this advice, but it can be very difficult to follow, even when the symptoms are quite disruptive.

> Never underestimate how a steady commitment to the broad principles of health can effect change.

Beyond these basics, much more detailed help and treatment plans are available, and I cover this process in the chapters in part III.

The figure overleaf shows just how interconnected the seven stress systems are. In the chapters in the next part, I explore in more detail the kinds of symptoms caused by activation of your seven stress systems, especially as these relate to pain and fatigue.

WHAT THE HELL IS WRONG WITH ME?

Your interactive seven stress systems in defensive mode

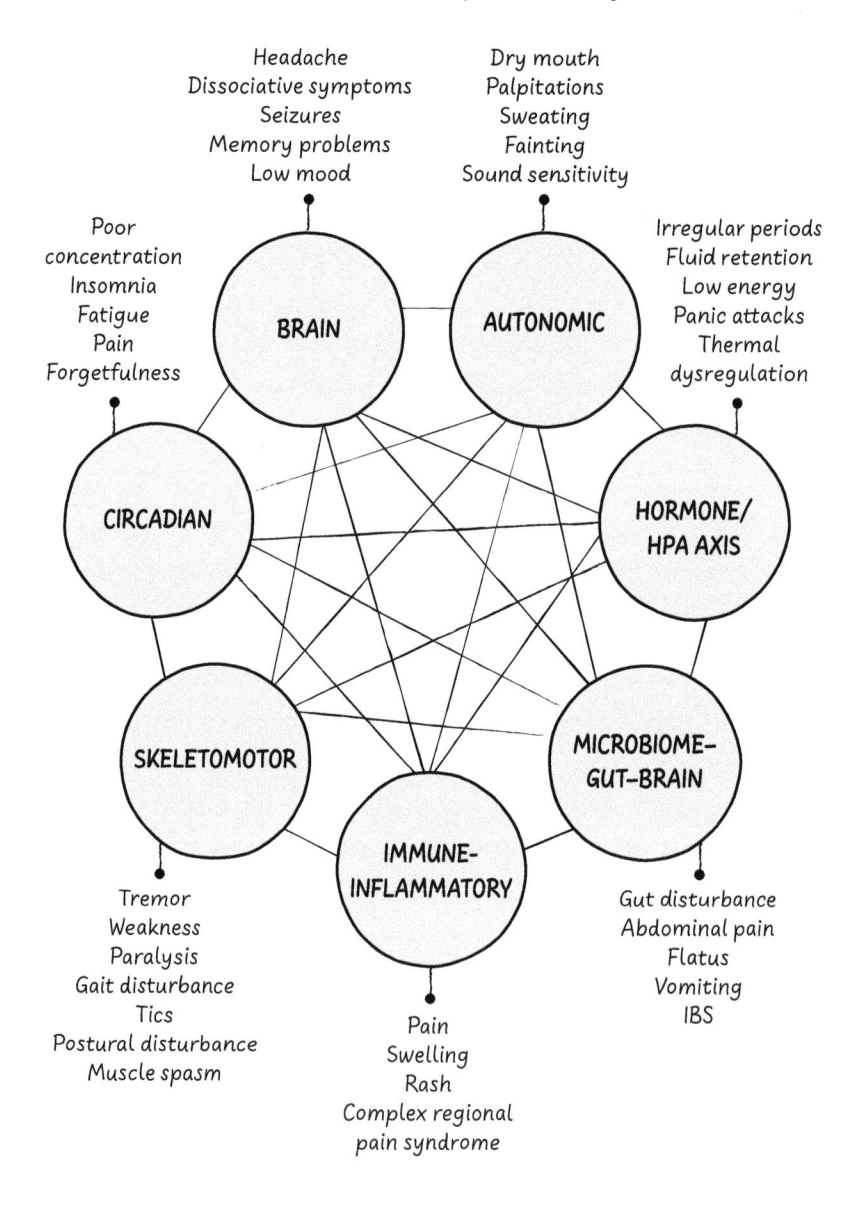

BRAIN
- Headache
- Dissociative symptoms
- Seizures
- Memory problems
- Low mood

AUTONOMIC
- Dry mouth
- Palpitations
- Sweating
- Fainting
- Sound sensitivity

CIRCADIAN
- Poor concentration
- Insomnia
- Fatigue
- Pain
- Forgetfulness

HORMONE/HPA AXIS
- Irregular periods
- Fluid retention
- Low energy
- Panic attacks
- Thermal dysregulation

SKELETOMOTOR
- Tremor
- Weakness
- Paralysis
- Gait disturbance
- Tics
- Postural disturbance
- Muscle spasm

IMMUNE-INFLAMMATORY
- Pain
- Swelling
- Rash
- Complex regional pain syndrome

MICROBIOME-GUT-BRAIN
- Gut disturbance
- Abdominal pain
- Flatus
- Vomiting
- IBS

Part II: Understanding pain, fatigue and the effect of negativity

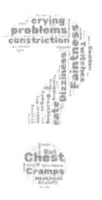

Chapter 5

A kaleidoscope of pain in functional disorders

I can't talk about functional conditions without exploring pain. Again, we have all had weird pains that come along. For most of us, these pains disappear as mysteriously as they came. For some of us, however, the pain stays and can even get worse. I'm not talking here about the obvious pain caused by injury or disease, which is often treatable, but the very troublesome and difficult-to-treat pain associated with functional conditions.

In this chapter, I delve into a deeper explanation of pain that exists without obvious cause – that is, functional pain syndromes.

Chronic versus acute pain

You no doubt understand what doctors call 'acute pain'. You stub your toe or burn yourself, for example, and experience some pain. You expect this pain to settle soon.

But you may have developed pain that continues without any obvious cause and fails to settle over weeks or months. Once you have had pain for more than three months, without an obvious cause such as a tumour or infection, doctors will often classify it as 'chronic pain'. We are now entering a difficult and distressing space. All the easily treatable causes of pain have been ruled out, but you continue to experience distressing levels of pain. Indeed, you get very little relief from even the strongest painkillers (which can make your pain worse). You seem to be running out of treatment options. None of the usual treatments seem to be working and you may sense a degree of pessimism when you keep reporting no improvement in your pain levels. Leila's story is an example of this.

LEILA

Leila came to see me three months after she had fallen onto her outstretched hand and fractured her wrist. Her surgeon was pleased with her recovery and told her the bone had healed after six weeks and she was free to use it normally. However, weeks on from the six-week mark, she was still not ready to give up her sling. I examined her arm and found it to be stiff and cold with wasted muscles. She winced when I tried to move her wrist, admitting that she was afraid it was not healed at all, based on her pain levels which were worse not better.

I double checked with her surgeon who confirmed her good outcome.

I knew that Leila's recovery would take a lot more than just time. Leila needed to understand what chronic pain was, if she had any chance of recovery, so let's go through this together.

Acute pain

When you hurt yourself – say, you step on a nail – you often feel pain immediately. The tissue damage caused by the nail triggers rapid nerve signals to the spine and a reflex reaction is triggered, often before you have conscious awareness of the injury. You might reflexively lift your foot off the nail. Your body tries to protect you, even without your choice.

Soon after this protective reflex, an inflammatory response starts. The injured cells release chemicals that alert the nearby nerves, and then the brain, to the extent of the problem, so you can consciously choose your next action, such as stop walking on that foot and, if safe, remove the nail.[14]

The local reaction also causes more blood to come to repair the injury, removing the damaged cells and associated debris. (When this reaction is strong, the area becomes red, swollen, and tender, and it can look like infection.)

The whole process happens locally, with the brain simply being informed of the progress, so it can dictate the early protective reflexes you might employ, such as nursing the area and only slowly returning to full use as the pain settles.

Almost all injuries heal this way within weeks. It is extraordinary how the body can repair itself so perfectly.

Chronic pain

However, when your pain experience is prolonged, like Leila's, other processes can arise that are far from perfect. In fact, when your pain becomes chronic, loosely considered to be around three months, your body might develop decidedly unhelpful responses. This chronic pain can then last for years without remission. It is a terrible and maladaptive response that serves no purpose other than to make us miserable. Mother Nature really lets us down here.

Chronic pain differs qualitatively from acute pain, often having a vague location and the potential to extend beyond the initial injury site. For instance, if you originally broke your wrist, the pain may now extend to your hand and arm, with altered sensations such as burning or stabbing. The pain also tends to be more relentless and severe than the initial pain, with even light touch feeling painful.

---

14 Interestingly, if your brain deems it is not safe to stop – for example, you are escaping from a burning house – it will not even let you feel pain, so you don't stop to remove the nail but keep running for your life. Only when it is safe will you become aware of the injury. How extraordinary is that?!

Doctors are still trying to understand what happens to cause this chronic pain and why only some people go on to develop this type of pain while others heal and recover, and also why some people (like Linus, mentioned in the introduction) just get pain out of the blue with no known cause.

What experts do know is that the brain is now receiving signals that the trauma or danger still exists, even though it doesn't; the pain is arising directly from the spinal cord and the neural pathways that generate pain in the brain. In other words, you may not have an injury, but you do have a pain problem.

In the previous chapter, I outlined the brain stress system, which is switched on when you experience a problem, such as an illness or injury, and switched off after the problem has healed. Experts now know from imaging studies of patients with chronic pain (and other functional conditions) that the brain stress systems fail to switch off, even though the danger has passed.

What happens instead is that the parts of your brain that make pain become hyperactive and can fire even with a stimulus as mild as light touch. Other stress systems activate too, such as the skeleto-motor system, which can cause weakness, and the autonomic nervous system, which can cause sweating and other nerve symptoms. Strange additional symptoms can also develop, and the pain can spread around the body, a long way from the initial site.

Ongoing activation of the brain stress systems uses a lot of energy and can lead to fatigue. If that wasn't enough, as covered in chapter 4, the stress system can turn on the immune-inflammatory system, which will make the pain worse by causing inflammation around the nerves. Macrophages, our wonderful little 'Pac-Man' cleaner cells, go feral and start causing inflammation throughout the body when the stress system is activated.

How to start a war

Imagine you have just developed a pain, out of nowhere, and you don't know what it is due to. Understandably, you may become stressed: what if it is a serious problem? What if it gets worse? You might start to imagine a full-blown catastrophe unfolding. Of course, you now know that your stress response system will respond to any threat, *real or imagined*, in the same way and activate every part of the system to defend you.

This is particularly true if you pay attention to a symptom. Focusing your mind on a symptom tends to exacerbate it and trigger a stronger stress response. Before you know it, your whole system is in defensive mode and a chain of interacting responses is playing havoc in your unsuspecting body: your brain stress system has intercepted the worrying thoughts and activated the defensive mode; the autonomic nervous system has immediately sprung into action, like a rapid response unit, and fired up the sympathetic nervous system; this has, in turn, released adrenaline, driving the skeletomotor system into a fight, flight or freeze response and tensing your body up for the imminent attack. Instead of healing, your circadian rhythm releases a flood of stress hormones which, in turn, drive up the inflammatory-immune system. Now your macrophages are spraying pro-inflammatory agents in readiness for the attack. The original pain may have gone, but you have set in motion a juggernaut of bodily responses that will continue to play out as long as the stress response systems are on. You are a wreck.

Fortunately, this doesn't happen every time you have a distressing thought or jab of pain, because you are also able to counter this thought with a judicious response. Your response to the pain, for example, may have been countered by a more philosophical attitude, or you may have been distracted by a joke or some tasks.

But, especially if you have a history of trauma, your systems can be on hair-trigger alert and that pain can be enough to set off World War III. (And remember, we don't yet know why this happens in some people.) When your stress systems have been activated too much – or too long or too little or simply fail to return to baseline – then functional symptoms like pain may arise. This may be why those with a history of trauma can remain unwell unless a deep level of healing takes place.

Enter chronic pain

As mentioned, with chronic pain, the brain's processing of messages becomes problematic. Understanding this is essential: when diagnosed with chronic pain syndrome, you need to modify your approach compared to managing acute pain. Recovery from chronic pain involves gradually restoring normal activity, tolerating pain while trusting that it will diminish with regained function.

> Remember – chronic pain can even occur in the absence of any physical injury, or long after the initial injury has healed.

That is, chronic pain is a functional disorder and to manage it, you need good information and a lot of support to find your way to recovery. Medication to modify the pain perception can be helpful.

The earlier you discover the real diagnosis of chronic pain, the faster you should recover. Unfortunately, a lot of people, including some doctors, fail to recognise the shift from acute to chronic pain and so continue to pursue acute pain treatments, with unfortunate results. Failing to return to using the injured body part, prolonged use of painkillers and feelings of anxiety or depression can aggravate the problem. Chronic pain is a source of massive social burden with poor outcomes, including failure to return to the workforce, ongoing suffering, and dependency on family and health services. We must do better.

So, let's go more deeply into the nature of chronic pain, because it is so common. It has been estimated that one in four Australians will experience chronic pain and many will never realise it.

Let's go back to Leila with her wrist fracture. She might understandably be worried that something is still wrong at the site of the injury, because that is what her brain was telling her. Leila needed to learn that the pain messages she was aware of were coming from her brain and not from her wrist. This took some convincing. In similar situations, your GP may need to turn to other health professionals for help.

Physiotherapists, for example, play a vital role in helping to safely restore full function. Note that modern physiotherapists can coach you to retrain your body and brain, through education and a range of exercises and activities. Their focus is on rehabilitation rather than excessive coddling, requiring you to work through some level of pain with the understanding that it is a necessary part of the recovery process. And you just need to trust the process.

The wonderful Australian pain specialist Professor Lorimer Moseley has developed some great material on this and other chronic pain conditions. For easily accessible information and resources to help you learn about pain-related conditions, I recommend the website of his organisation Pain Revolution – www.painrevolution.org. Professor Moseley's insights and treatments are of enormous help – also check out his YouTube talks (details provided in appendix C) because he is able to convey the complex and difficult ideas about chronic pain in a clever, entertaining and even funny way. (Who would have thought chronic pain could be funny?!)

The experience of chronic pain can be worse and more disabling than the original pain, and it requires a distinct approach and perspective for management. Medication to modify pain perception can be helpful, but early diagnosis of chronic pain is crucial for a faster recovery. Education, support and rehabilitation will help you manage your chronic pain. You may need your doctor, pain psychologist and physiotherapist to help with your recovery.

Complex regional pain syndrome

You may have noticed that Leila didn't simply have pain. She also had visible changes in her arm, which was stiff, wasted and clammy. She had a particular type of chronic pain, called 'complex regional pain syndrome'.

Complex regional pain syndrome (CRPS) can occur anywhere but is particularly likely to occur in the limbs, following an injury or surgery. Instead of the pain settling, with this syndrome you might notice increased pain, burning or stabbing sensations, and a strong disinclination to use the limb, which may become cooler, clammier, more swollen and stiffer than the opposite limb.

Experts don't understand why some people develop this nasty condition. But they are beginning to know how to manage it and, especially if diagnosed early, we can achieve a great outcome.

One of the most important discoveries about CRPS is that the messages from the limb to the brain are altered en route. Instead of feeling normal touch, for example, a person with CRPS will feel pain. Another way to say this is that the pain is not coming from the limb; instead, it is coming from the nerves, including the autonomic nerves, the spinal cord and the pain centres in the brain.

In order to recover from CRPS, you need to overcome the instinctive response to pain (keep immobile and protected), and learn to accept and work through the pain to achieve a good outcome. Medication can help to dampen the unhelpful pain messages but, in the end, people with CRPS need to develop a trusting relationship with their healthcare providers to get the support they need to recover. Sometimes, CRPS patients will need to work with psychologists, physiotherapists, pain specialists, GPs and occupational therapists to facilitate recovery.

> **REPETITIVE STRAIN INJURY**
>
> In chapter 2 I include the role of sociocultural influences on functional conditions and mention the 'Beatlemania' that many young women experienced in the early 1960s. An egregious

example of this influence is the remarkable rise and fall of what came to be known as repetitive strain injury or RSI.

The new phenomenon of arm pain, sometimes affecting whole typing pools, arose in epidemic proportions in Australia in the 1980s and threatened to overwhelm the workers compensation system.

Despite millions of dollars of research, no evidence of injury was ever found in these patients. It is important to differentiate RSI from other occupational overuse syndromes with identifiable physical injuries, such as tendonitis or carpal tunnel syndrome, which have a recognised pattern of symptoms and physical signs and a reasonably predictable response to treatment. However, despite no physical cause, RSI patients suffered real pain and were often unable to continue their work.

RSI patients had pain in a diffuse pattern, not localised to any particular muscle or nerve. So calling it an injury is probably inaccurate. It was a regional pain syndrome, a functional condition, which arose in a particular sociocultural group of vulnerable workers. These days, it has largely disappeared, even though the work conditions that led to it are still occurring. It has not been proven that the changes in work practices, such as better ergonomics, controlled rates of typing and increased work breaks, made a difference in the epidemic settling.

The outbreak of RSI illustrates how certain social groups can develop health problems in the context of certain technological changes, societal pressures and work conditions, and that the condition can appear to spread like an infection throughout the social group.

The huge controversy over the cause and even the very existence of symptoms typifies the struggle experienced by sufferers of functional conditions. The range of responses within the medical profession to the surprising surge in cases of (mainly) women with disabling arm pain reflected the attitude rather than the skills of the doctors. Everything from sympathy to well-meaning and contradictory advice to outright disbelief would be proffered. It remains unclear what led to the surge and people still develop similar symptoms but more as individual cases.

> In the case of RSI, nicknamed Kangaroo Paw, Australia gained worldwide notoriety for the dramatic rise and eventual fall of RSI without there being any sign of injury. Many sufferers were able to return to the same work without further symptoms.

The predictive processing model

Remember Kirralee from chapter 4, who would wake with a whole lot of terrifying symptoms that made her fear for her life? To further understand what happened to Kirralee, and what turned her normal day into a terrifying health scare, we need to understand some more concepts.

Scientists used to think the brain was like a computer. We feed in some data or stimulus, and it churns out a response. And this is partly true.

But a whole other system is also at work. As we grow, we humans learn, through trial and error or through learnt knowledge, that certain events can be predicted. We can anticipate these events and automatically set up a response in readiness. For example, from experience, we know that a hot drink can burn our lips, so we reflexively blow on the drink or sip very slowly to test the temperature. Another example is automatically ducking when a loud sound goes off. We anticipate, using our predictive processing, that a loud sound could be accompanied by a flying object that could hurt us, so we duck. All good so far.

But some predictive processing is unhelpful. A rubber snake joke would never work without predictive processing. We leap out of our skin on seeing a snake on our path, only to have the joker pick up the rubber toy, laughing at our expense. The joker relied on us having learned 'snakes are dangerous' and responding to the supposed threat by leaping into the air. The predictive processing model is an automatic, subconscious bodily defence system – and it is a common source of functional symptoms.

As Kirralee's story shows, while the predictive processing model can help us to avoid injury, it can also lead to unhelpful responses.

Although as an adult Kirralee had secured a safe home, far away from the place of her childhood traumas, her predictive processing set off the alarms and she found herself seemingly under attack once more. But this time, she was not fending off physical attacks; her brain had reacted to 'night-time' as if a threat was imminent and triggered a panic attack. Kirralee was unaware of the role of predictive processing in her sudden symptoms; she just thought that her heart was about to stop under the strain. It is understandable why she felt this.

Kirralee's nightmarish panic attacks stemmed from childhood experiences that ingrained in her subconscious the belief that 'bad things happen at night'. Her middle-of-the-night awakenings with rapid palpitations were not consciously linked to her childhood trauma. According to the predictive processing model, as Kirralee tried to sleep, her subconscious memories activated her brain stress system, triggering the belief that 'nights are when you can be attacked'. Consequently, her defensive mode was activated in her subconscious mind, triggering all her symptoms.

Her brain stress system only then consciously identifies the effect of the hyperventilation and increased heart rate and senses a full-blown stress situation, triggering thoughts of serious health problems causing panic and fear, thereby increasing the flood of stress hormones and turning on a full fight, flight or freeze response.

This process is shown in the figure overleaf.

Eventually, by working with her psychologist and regulating her autonomic nervous system with her osteopath, Kirralee was able to recognise her anxiety, previously essential for survival, was now unwarranted. This meant she was able to override her defensive mode and regain her calm restorative mode.

Unconscious stressors can cause conscious panic

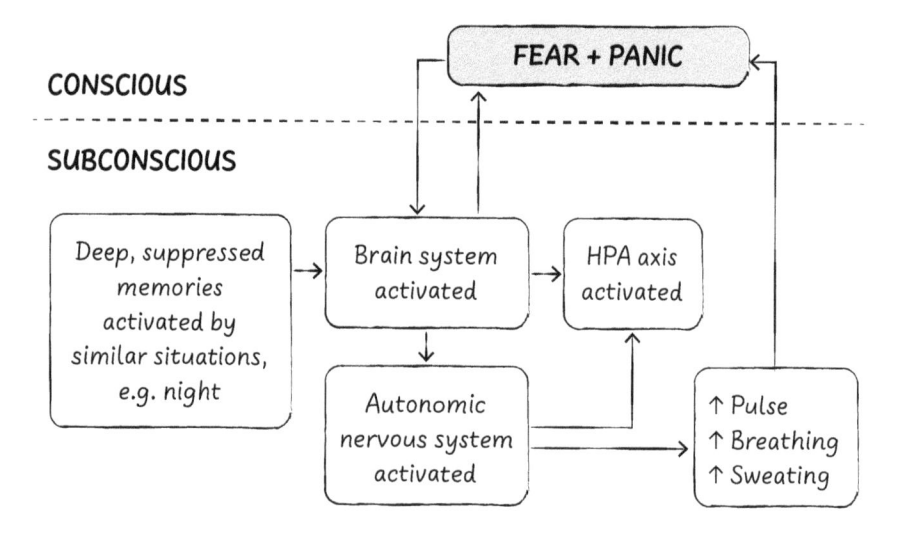

```
                          ┌─────────────┐
CONSCIOUS                 │ FEAR + PANIC│ ←───┐
                          └─────────────┘     │
- - - - - - - - - - - - - - - -↑- - - - - - - │ - -
SUBCONSCIOUS                   │               │
                               │               │
┌──────────────┐   ┌──────────────┐   ┌──────────────┐
│Deep,suppressed│→ │ Brain system │ → │   HPA axis   │
│   memories   │   │  activated   │   │  activated   │
│ activated by │   └──────────────┘   └──────────────┘
│similar situations│      ↓                   ↑
│  e.g. night  │   ┌──────────────┐   ┌──────────────┐
└──────────────┘   │  Autonomic   │   │ ↑ Pulse      │
                   │nervous system│ → │ ↑ Breathing  │
                   │  activated   │   │ ↑ Sweating   │
                   └──────────────┘   └──────────────┘
```

> Remember – throughout whatever illness you have, you need to continue to report any new developments in your symptoms to your doctor. People with functional conditions can get physical illnesses too, of course. And many people with pre-existing physical illnesses can develop functional symptoms as well. If you notice that things have progressed and you find yourself seeking medical attention, be reassured that that is exactly what you should do.

Examples of recurring and chronic pain

Chronic pain can manifest in many different ways. In the following sections, I run through some of the more common.

Headache

While the causes of headache are vast, most of them have normal findings – that is, they are functional. Indeed, mostly the diagnosis can be made without the need for tests or scans.

Because headaches are so common, a lot is known about them and how to treat them. Of course, the best action is prevention, which requires attention to all the factors that contribute to their development. I find a lot of headache sufferers are not aware of their triggers – for example, poor posture or muscle tension, such as happens with teeth-grinding.

For some, different types of headache can coexist, such as tension headaches and migraine. It is always a good idea to bring your headache diary to your doctor's appointment so they can estimate how much your life is affected and how effective your treatment is.

Another helpful approach to headache is to take time to observe how you live in your body, what demands you place upon yourself or allow others to, and what you do when your body requires attention, such as hydration or even rest. Start paying kind attention to your body's needs before it is screaming at you with pain.

Some people are terrified that they have a serious problem such as a brain tumour and cannot believe that frequent or serious pain can be 'just functional'. Of course, the stress of such fear can add to the headache problem. But you may notice a pattern in your headache intensity or frequency with changes in the demands upon you – for example, when you have a really good break from life's demands. Serious medical conditions do not pay much heed to these changes.

For further help in this area, the Australia and New Zealand Headache Society (anzheadachesociety.org) provides a lot of useful information, including a good diary template. More resources are available in appendix C.

Back pain

The experience of back pain is almost universal but, for some, it is a source of ongoing misery. Your doctor can rule out the medical causes of back pain, using the Red Flag method described later.

But if you think about your body as a machine, then you might think that pain is due to something damaged that should be repaired. This is not always a helpful thought. Just like with headaches, many simple measures can be done while the back pain settles. The general advice is to continue light activity, if possible, and allow time for the pain to settle, as it generally does over days.

But if, for example, you react to the unpleasant pains with fear that you have a serious injury, you might aggravate the problem with undue worries and stress. Having read this far, you will realise that the body stress system can activate back problems, by triggering your immune-inflammatory response or even involuntarily tensing your muscles through your skeletomotor activation.

Other beliefs can also make it likely the back pain will persist or even get worse. Once fearful beliefs arise, you likely find it difficult to move normally and restore function. If you believe that every pain is a result of more damage, your return to normal activity is likely to be hampered. In chapter 13, I look more into the effect of belief systems and other non-medical factors that can affect your recovery and what you can do about them.

Whiplash

Having your head violently thrown about, typically in an accident, will quite likely lead to strains and sprains of any number of muscles and ligaments in your neck, as well as the tendons attached to your spine. You may suffer from dizziness and headaches and find it difficult to do the most basic things afterwards.

Fortunately, for most people, these nasty symptoms will ease over days to weeks. But for some people, the symptoms will linger and be a cause of considerable distress. In this case, it is advisable to be examined by a doctor so you can be confident your movements will not cause more harm. While analgesics and physiotherapy certainly can aid recovery, it is helpful to engage a psychologist who understands the disruptive and frightening aspects of your condition and can support you in your efforts to recover. Once again, this is not to say that your symptoms are simply psychological. (To find out more about all the things your psychologist can assist you with, see chapter 13.)

Chest pain

As stated repeatedly in this book, chest pain is something that doctors take seriously every time, no matter what was diagnosed previously. That is because if the source of pain is the heart or other vital organs such as the lungs, prompt treatment is necessary. While causes of chest pain can come from other organs or the spine, chest pain is a relatively common functional symptom, because the chest is where the stress response plays out. Remember Kirralee's panicked emergency dashes to the hospital from chapter 4? Her attending hospital was appropriate, but it took a long time for her to establish that her chest tightness and pains were functional.

Ear pain

Patients commonly request antibiotics for an ear infection, only for me to find no sign of any inflammation that would suggest an infection.

But pressure on the anterior (front) of the offending ear canal might reproduce the pain, making it likely that the pain is due to temporomandibular joint dysfunction. Once again, tests are normal but the patient has lots of pain.

Releasing the tension in the jaw muscles can bring relief. Sometimes, the tight muscles are in the back of the mouth. A good physiotherapist can find the culprit and – hey presto! Relief!

Botox injections are sometimes necessary if the clenching occurs during sleep, because this can lead to a depressing cycle of pain, clenching as a response to pain, leading to further pain.

Referred pain

Referred pain is pain that is felt at a different location from where it arises. Many people know that sciatica is pain in the leg caused by a problem in the spine – that is, sciatica is a referred pain. However, referred pain is a common source of confusion when chest pain arises.

Chest pain can be referred from the muscles on the chest wall. Even people who have previously experienced true cardiac pain, or a heart attack, can mistake chest wall pain for more heart trouble. This is one more oddity about pain: the brain holds the memory of the serious pain from the heart attack, but when a pain arises from a nearby structure, it sometimes misinterprets it as the same as the heart attack pain.

Another example of this misattribution of pain is Jinni's story.

JINNI

Jinni woke one morning to a nasty pain in her lower right abdomen. As it continued to get worse, she went to hospital and was diagnosed with appendicitis. Following her appendicectomy, she made a quick recovery. But a few months later, she again developed abdominal pain and had the exact same symptoms. She knew it couldn't be her appendix, but it felt just the same. I treated her for constipation and her 'appendicitis' pain settled.

So, when you feel pain, you can attribute it with great conviction to the wrong thing. Jinni was able to easily accept it was not her appendix (because she no longer had one) but doctors often struggle to convince their patients about other misattributions – for example, that their chest pain is not coming from the heart. It is totally understandable that you might want to say something like, 'I know what I feel and it is definitely my heart.' Keeping in mind that other body protection system, the predictive processing model (outlined earlier in this chapter), can help with understanding the nature of pain interpretation.

Breast pain

Similarly, breast pain can also arise from the chest wall and not the breast. I often have to demonstrate that the breast itself is not tender, but the chest wall under the breast is the source of pain. Once your breast examination (perhaps with mammogram and/or ultrasound) is normal, you can seek relief from your physiotherapist.

Pelvic pain

Functional symptoms can arise in the pelvis and mimic physical problems such as urinary tract infections or endometriosis.

This type of functional pain can coexist with physical disorders, making diagnosis difficult, because we cannot rely on the symptoms alone. In these patients, I test to exclude infection every time. For those with coexisting endometriosis, working with a good pelvic physiotherapist, along with some pain-modifying medication, can make a big difference.

Pelvic pain is more common in women who have had sexual assaults and this is not necessarily due to direct physical effects. Why pain can arise without a physical cause is not clear.

Psychological support and, importantly, validation of your pain experience without necessarily attributing it to endometriosis, and identifying possible triggers are all important. It is surprising how a very tense pelvic floor muscle can mimic pain from other previously affected pelvic organs. Esther's story is an example of this.

ESTHER

Esther would present every now and then requesting antibiotics for what she thought was a urinary tract infection. The problem was that the urine never showed any signs of infection. We would debate the management and it took me quite a while to persuade Esther that her symptoms were actually due to pelvic floor dysfunction, where her muscles would tighten into discomfort, increasing to painful spasms during the passing of urine. Pelvic floor physiotherapy to release the tension proved effective and Esther had no further symptoms.

Again, functional symptoms can mimic, or at least be interpreted by the mind as representing, a known condition. Esther had been convinced she had an infection, because her brain interpreted the muscle spasm to be just like the remembered pain of an infected bladder.

Myofascial pain syndrome

'Myalgia' is the word for pain in your muscles. This can occur with injury and other causes, but sometimes you can have pain and all your tests are normal. The pain is localised to a particular area (as opposed to fibromyalgia, discussed in the next section). Common places where you might experience myofascial pain are across the shoulders or neck. It can be tender to press on. These tender knots are called trigger points. Interestingly, the pain can be felt elsewhere when you press on the trigger point. For example, if you have a trigger point in a neck muscle, it can 'radiate' down the arm. As pain going down the arm can be a symptom of a heart attack, this can precipitate a trip to hospital.

The features of myofascial pain are sometimes poorly understood by doctors, except with specific conditions such as tension headache. But muscles are a very common source of functional pain and can respond wonderfully to the correct diagnosis and treatment. Physiotherapists, on the other hand, are dab at recognising these trigger points and treating them.

So, pain anywhere from the top of your head to your big toe can be, and most commonly is, due to myofascial pain.

Fibromyalgia

Fibromyalgia also includes muscle pain but is a different entity. Here the aches and pains are widespread, often symmetrical, and associated with fatigue, unrefreshing sleep and feeling unwell.

Once again, you should be investigated for physical diseases, but it is more common for these tests to be normal.

Imagine waking every morning, feeling like you have a bad case of flu – every morning with no relief. This is the lived experience for those with fibromyalgia, a classic example of a functional disorder, where despite widespread symptoms, all tests are normal.

Once again, experts don't know what causes fibromyalgia, but prolonged periods of poor-quality sleep are a frequent finding. Whether this is the cause or simply one of the symptoms is still under debate. It is a condition that will often persevere for months if not treated. For more information, look in Resources in appendix C.

The widespread aches make the sufferer feel like physical activity is the last thing they want to do, but for recovery to happen, a graded program of increasing physical activity is often helpful.

Another symptom experienced by fibromyalgia sufferers is uncommonly frequent and severe fatigue. The nature and chronicity of fibromyalgia distinctly overlaps with persistent fatigue syndrome, with some unfortunate folk experiencing high levels of both muscle aches and fatigue. I look into fatigue and its mysteries in the next chapter.

Chapter 6

Beyond exhaustion: Navigating the labyrinth of fatigue in functional disorders

Fatigue is one of the most frustrating symptoms to have, and it is also one of the common reasons people visit their GP. About one in five people seeing their GP give tiredness as their reason. It deserves its own exploration because it is such a common symptom – and that's what this chapter is all about.

Defining fatigue

Fatigue is complex: it is one of the main symptoms of many diseases. Only when all these have been excluded is the functional condition of persistent fatigue diagnosed. Fatigue can occur at any age and seemingly without reason. It is hard to describe. And yet, fatigue is often a disabling symptom. It can prevent you from doing your normal activities, lead you to miss out on so many things, and ruin your plans.

Fatigue also means different things to people; for example, someone may say fatigue but mean muscle weakness or a lack of motivation and interest or sleepiness. Doctors consider fatigue to mean exhaustion that doesn't go away after rest, lack of energy, tiredness, difficulty thinking or heaviness of the limbs.

One of the features of fatigue is that it is purely subjective – there is no way to measure or see fatigue. People with fatigue can do things if they have to – for example, escape a dangerous situation – but it would take a superhuman effort. There is no actual muscle weakness when tested, and sufferers seem to be getting enough sleep but wake up as if they did not sleep much at all.

Doctors are adept at excluding the usual medical conditions that cause fatigue and will start with your history, asking questions such as the following:

- When did the fatigue first appear?
- Are there any other symptoms?
- Is it present every day?
- Are there aggravating and ameliorating factors?

If fatigue is truly the only symptom, identifying a disease is difficult, because most diseases have other symptoms. But, your answers to this line of questioning help your doctor to exclude certain conditions, and it is usual to do a complete physical examination, some office tests and then order some blood investigations. This is a good place to start. It might surprise you to know that most of these tests usually come back normal – except for low iron levels, which is quite common.

Yet, what can be more disappointing than undergoing a battery of tests to investigate your fatigue, only for them all to be frustratingly normal?

Once assured that your physical examination and tests are normal, your doctor at this stage will often employ the time-honoured strategy of 'watchful expectation' – that is, careful observation matched with masterly inactivity on the part of the doctor will often bring the desired outcome: recovery. Another way to say this is the old saying, 'time heals' – except, of course, it sometimes needs help.

Your healthcare team can also turn their efforts towards addressing those factors that could be contributing to your fatigue. The syndrome of persistent fatigue is described as when you have had fatigue for more than six months. In other words, having some fatigue following a demanding period in your life or after an illness is common, but most people recover eventually. People with persistent fatigue just don't. This is when you and your healthcare team need to focus your attention on every single factor that could cause ordinary fatigue and every single effort that could be helpful to lift your fatigue right now.

Sleep deprivation

Sleep deprivation is such a common problem these days that many people fail to recognise this obvious source of tiredness – and its effect. (As sleep expert Ryan Hurd notes, 'Sleep deprivation is an illegal torture method outlawed by the Geneva Convention and international courts, but most of us do it to ourselves.') But, as I outline in chapter 4, the effects of inadequate sleep are profound, so it is a good place to start checking for the reasons for your tiredness.

As housing affordability is driving workers further from their place of employment, the longer commuting times are eating into a balanced lifestyle of the famous 'Eight hours labour, eight hours recreation, eight hours rest' proposed by labour advocate Robert Owen over 200 years ago.

Of course, many working women come home from their place of employment, only to have to do the housework and caregiving, disproportionately doing more than their male partners. Add in waking in the night to care for sick children or looking after aged parents and the levels of fatigue become overwhelming.

Sleep quality is as important as quantity

As anyone who has tried to sleep while travelling can testify, you can wake up fatigued even if you seem to have been sleeping for hours. But, due to the invention of sleep laboratories, we now know how important it is to get good-quality sleep. Many factors can interfere with sleep quality. An over-busy mind, stimulant drugs such as caffeine, PTSD, a noisy environment, pain, depression and anxiety, and obstructive sleep apnoea can all lead to a reduction in the amount of deep, restorative sleep.

If you are fatigued, a useful starting point is to simply record how much sleep you are getting. People who are wearing recording devices can get some idea how much deep, restorative sleep they are getting. This information is very helpful to determine if there is a simple cause for your fatigue.

Given the significant impact of not getting enough good-quality sleep, this needs to be given proper attention. Relying on neurostimulants during waking hours, such as caffeine and other drugs, is no substitute for a good night's sleep. For more information and tips on how to improve your sleep quantity and quality, see chapter 14.

Other common causes of fatigue

Getting enough good-quality sleep may be only one side of the equation. In the following sections, I outline other factors that may be contributing to your fatigue.

Food, fads, fasting and fatigue

Another often overlooked source of fatigue is a neglected diet. In medical school, we studied the role of every single chemical needed to keep the body running smoothly, and what struck me was the need for every mitochondrion (cellular power pack) in every one of the 100 trillion cells in the body to have an adequate supply of vitamins, minerals, proteins and lipids (fats) to work. What happens when these nutrients aren't available? The body simply cannot do its work properly and you feel like your body is struggling to function – that is, it is fatigued. This is simply a fact of life. For more on how to get enough of the essential nutrients in your diet, see chapter 14.

Unrealistic expectations

Have you ever known someone who drives themselves relentlessly and then cannot accept that their body protests with extreme fatigue levels? It is like their mind, with its unrealistic ambitions, is a ruthless slavedriver demanding a punishing schedule of work, until the enslaved body drops from fatigue. The mind responds only with more flogging, forcing the body to continue without proper rest until it collapses completely. Maree's crippling fatigue, which I outline in chapter 8, was partially due to this.

I find energy supplies vary greatly and some people have an extraordinary capacity for work, slogging on for hours without flagging, while others operate best with short bursts of exertion before a rest is needed for best functioning.

The ancient Indian system of health, Ayurvedic medicine, has described these qualities in detail, recognising the vastly different types of human functioning that exists. This approach views physical wellbeing as being interdependent with emotional and spiritual wellbeing, and uses treatments such as yoga, meditation, dietary changes and herbal medicines to treat the causes of ill health. I recommend a visit to an Ayurvedic practitioner if your doctor assures you there is no medical reason for your fatigue. It can be very liberating to recognise and work within your naturally determined limits, rather than some arbitrary social or family expectations.

As an aside, while many doctors suffer from workaholism, this is not seen as a virtue, nor is it necessarily sustainable. Overwork can lead to all manner of mental health problems, but fixating on the work issues can blind you to the real issue of energy imbalance: supply and demand need to be kept even if you are to keep going and sustain your health.

What has happened to the eight-hour day?

Workers have long fought for better work conditions, and principal among these are restricted hours of labour. As early as the sixteenth century King Philip II of Spain, by royal edict, declared the eight-hour day.

But the Industrial Revolution, which swept first through Great Britain and then Europe and the United States in the eighteenth and nineteenth centuries, drove men, women and children into factories, often working 12 to 16 hours, with only one day's respite a week. Karl Marx observed this and wrote in *Das Kapital* (1867):

> *By extending the working day, therefore, capitalist production ... not only produces a deterioration of human labour-power by robbing it of its normal, moral and physical, conditions of development and activity but also produces the premature exhaustion and death of this labour-power itself.*

Eventually, news of the horrific deaths of children (after dropping asleep and falling into the machinery) helped lead to industrial reform.

Australia should be proud that it led the industrial world by achieving the eight-hour day in the 1850s for some workers. It took a while for the world to catch on, but those advances are now being undermined by modern working practices. In theory, the working week is meant to be 38 hours, but since COVID, a lot of unpaid overtime is being done which undermines the long-established healthy working hours. The result is fatigue.

Humans can put up with such stressors for a long time, but it can lead to changes in mental health. Three conditions that are common sources of fatigue are burnout, anxiety and depression.

Burnout

Burnout is recognised as a syndrome attributed to ongoing stressors in the workplace that have not been well managed. According to the World Health Organization (WHO), burnout has three elements:

1. feelings of energy depletion or exhaustion
2. increased mental distance from one's job, or feelings of negativism or cynicism related to one's job
3. reduced professional efficacy.

In the industrial world, burnout is a common phenomenon. And a weekend off just is not enough to address the psychic and physical stressors that have been probably accumulating over months. Seeking support and talking to others (including your boss) is a vital first step.[15]

> **THE CHICKEN AND THE EGG**
>
> What if your fatigue is attributed to your drinking too much alcohol? Yes, maybe, but what has driven you to drink? The extra demands of work? The lack of control over your job expectations? Poor work–life balance? The need for self-soothing?
>
> Before any judgement is made about the causes of any harmful drinking, a broader perspective about the issues affecting your life and your response to them is helpful. In chapter 11, I take a look at the most beneficial approach to take when dealing with a complex tangle of symptoms and external factors.

Mental health and fatigue

Anyone trying to live with disabling fatigue would naturally feel depressed so another chicken-and-egg situation exists here: did the fatigue cause the depression or vice versa? Regardless of the answer, we have to work on whatever we can to help.

If you have ever suffered from anxiety or depression, you would be aware of how fatiguing it is. My patients have described the fatigue as like walking through molasses, or told of the superhuman

---

[15] For more information on the causes and costs of burnout, and some tips on how to recover from it, see the Mayo Clinic's article 'Job burnout: How to spot it and take action' (www.mayoclinic.org/healthy-lifestyle/adult-health/in-depth/burnout/art-20046642).

effort required just to get out of bed in the morning. That they continue to work despite these struggles is remarkable.

The huge amount of nervous energy used to navigate the stressful reactions that occur in the anxious mind is like spending the whole day running up a hill, with little respite. Mental health problems just drain the batteries. And because sleep is often disturbed too, there is no revival overnight. The inefficiencies of the stressed mind make work very difficult, and every task takes a lot more effort. It is hardly surprising that the fatigue associated with anxiety is so crippling.

Depression can be even more fatiguing. I have seen patients so deeply depressed that they do not have the means to eat or even talk. Depression is not a functional condition, but severely disabling fatigue can be due to an underlying mental illness.

However, it is not uncommon for people to fail to recognise their own decline in mental health and instead focus on either perceived excessive demands from external sources or perhaps a fear of some physical condition. I once had a patient who had moved house eight times, thinking her accommodation was the cause of her being unwell and fatigued. When she eventually let me treat her depression, her energy returned and, to her husband's infinite relief, they stopped moving. She had been so focused on the things she usually achieved and then couldn't that she did not notice the general slide in her mood or increasing stress levels. A careful mental health history can help. A quick and easy way to check your mental health immediately is via an online quiz on a reputable website, such as BeyondBlue – go to www.beyondblue.org.au and click the 'I want to check my mental health' link.

Hiding in plain sight

Have you ever felt the need to talk to someone about a problem, but found yourself struggling to find the right words so you end up just saying that you are tired? Maybe you even find it hard to admit what is going on for you. Dorothy was like this when she first came to see me.

DOROTHY

I could see that Dorothy was not her usual ebullient self from the moment she came into the surgery. She sat slumped in the chair and clearly was having trouble describing the reason she had come. 'I'm just not feeling myself, I guess,' she said vaguely. I waited for her to expand on this and after a long pause, she ventured that things were not quite right at home. She was tired and did not feel like doing the things she used to do. 'I'm just so tired …' Another long pause. This was not leading anywhere quickly and yet it was obvious that something was troubling this usually cheerful mother of two. 'I'm probably being silly, and I know Charles is working very late these days. I'm often asleep when he comes home. But it has been months since we were … intimate.' She paused, and then said, 'Charles thinks that I should have a check-up, you know, blood tests and things.' I duly went ahead with this but knew that we were still wide of the mark. When she came back and was told all the results were normal, she seemed not to react. But suddenly she said, almost as an aside, 'I found some earrings in his pocket, you know. Quite flashy – not like the ones I wear.' She winced and looked away.

Doctors know that difficult issues such as domestic violence, gambling, or sexual or financial worries can present with socially acceptable symptoms such as fatigue. However, many a doctor has missed this cue to explore these difficult areas. Doctors generally try to be open to whatever problem is current, but this is a delicate forum because patients can be highly incensed when their doctor enquires about such taboo topics.

ALAN

Alan was just 18 when he came to see me about his longstanding fatigue. He had suffered from exhaustion and poor concentration since early in high school and had needed to drop out and study remotely for the previous two years. He was fortunate that this coincided with the remote teaching established during the COVID lockdown. But he missed all the sport and the normal socialising of a teenager.

Alan had undergone extensive testing, which helped to rule out most known physical conditions. He had gained height and weight as expected and his physical findings were satisfactory.

Because his fatigue levels hadn't improved, we agreed it was time to engage a psychologist.

What surprised Alan were the results of his anxiety testing. He was quite a lot younger when he had first been assessed and I suspect that at the time Alan did not have the language to describe his difficulties and felt more comfortable calling it tiredness and fatigue, rather than anxiety.

He worked on addressing the cause of his anxiety with his new psychologist and went on to regain a state of calm he had long forgotten and, with it, a restoration of his energy.

Did Alan suffer from persistent fatigue, or did he suffer from crippling levels of anxiety?

Persistent fatigue

If you have ongoing fatigue, you should undergo a thorough search for the cause, including mental conditions such as anxiety or depression. But, as discussed, fatigue can sometimes be present when all tests appear normal. If it persists for more than six months without a cause being found, you and your healthcare team need to consider the possibility of a functional cause.

Experts still have much to learn about persistent fatigue, and I am not suggesting that all undiagnosed fatigue is functional. Yet, without a better solution, you may benefit from determining whether your body stress systems (as outlined in chapter 4) have been activated, and then focusing on the means to settle them.

If you have the kinds of symptoms outlined in this chapter and in chapter 4, it is helpful to get a definite diagnosis from a knowledgeable doctor. (Unfortunately, some members of the medical community still struggle with a diagnosis for which there is no known test.) The reason it is beneficial to receive a positive diagnosis early is that you can confirm that the necessary medical investigations and mental health assessments are normal, so the management can then be focused on what experts in this area know are the most effective ways to lead to recovery. Early diagnosis and treatment will lead to a good recovery in most patients. (This contrasts with those who are not given the same level of support and whose symptoms may continue for years unabated.)

> Managing your expectations in terms of what you can and cannot do is a critical part of your recovery.

It might be helpful to use the Karnofsky Performance Scale[16] to help you estimate your expected recovery time. You can usually expect to recover 10 per cent of your activity levels each year.

'My brain has gone AWOL'

Problems with memory and concentration are part of many functional conditions, when the brain stress system is disrupted. You may have found yourself unable to remember the names of friends and family, or your academic or work performance has declined. Just the act of speaking, reading or writing can be difficult.

This is a frightening problem and only serves to make you feel worse. You may wonder if you will ever recover your mental capacity. Some people start googling the symptoms of dementia and see alarming similarities. It is important that you talk to your doctor

---

16 To access this scale, go to www.mdcalc.com/calc/3168/karnofsky-performance-status-scale.

about your fears and concerns. Having feelings of terror and hopelessness accompanying a belief that you have dementia will make it difficult for you to recover.

The good news is that (unlike those with true dementia) most people with a disrupted brain stress system due to a functional disorder do make a good recovery in both their fatigue levels and their mental capacity.

So, what do the experts know about the reasons that your brain is not functioning normally with persistent fatigue? It is still an area of much research, but let's focus on what happens in your brain when you have an activated brain stress system.

Firstly, as anyone who has ever had a bad night's sleep knows, good-quality sleep is essential for your brain to work well. I explore the role of disturbed sleep in chapter 4, but it is worth reiterating the main message: if your brain stress system has been turned on and is unable to be turned off, your sleep cycle and restorative functions of a healthy circadian rhythm will be disrupted. Night after night of poor sleep leads to a cycle of daytime mental under-functioning. Very little is good about this, except one thing: your brain itself is going to be fine when you find your way back to health. So, don't despair. In chapter 14, I outline how to return to that vital state, your restorative mode, and make use of its capacity to repair damage and remove debris that is essential for normal brain functioning.

A chronic state of activated defensive mode causes disturbance in cortisol levels via activation of your hypothalamic–pituitary–adrenal axis. It's like the rabbit-in-a-spotlight situation: your brain can't function on a higher, executive level. Executive functions of the brain include planning, keeping focus even when distractions arise, ordering priorities, meeting goals and displaying self-control. Without these functions, your brain cannot complete its usual tasks.

All the while you remain in defensive mode, through your hormone system you have increased levels of stress hormones (noradrenalin, endogenous opioids, endogenous cannabinoids, and other anaesthetic neurochemicals) that are secreted as part of the brain's stress response during states of high arousal. These stress hormones likewise disturb functioning in the executive regions of the brain. I outline the adverse effects of remaining in the fight, flight or freeze state in chapter 4. Remember that this state can be so persistent that it is hardly recognised, especially in the mental fog of persistent fatigue.

Chronic or episodic hyperventilation plays a role in disrupting mental functioning, as we highlighted in chapter 4. Unlike the dramatic events experienced by Ethan, ongoing mild hyperventilation and the consequent low levels of brain carbon dioxide cause brain fog. And yet, in persistent fatigue, it is very difficult to use physical activity to restore normal levels.

Study in this area is ongoing (see following section), and researchers will uncover more reasons why the function of your brain is reduced during persistent fatigue. But is it any wonder that with all these disruptions to your normal mental working, you are finding it hard to use your brain?

Present areas of research

Experts still have a lot to learn about functional conditions and research continues in areas such as neuroscience and the study of the brain, using imaging such as functional MRIs. The use of this new technology has been extremely interesting in helping us understand the neurological processes that occur during functional neurological disorders. A functional MRI can show which part of the brain is reacting during episodes. As an example, MRIs of subjects with functional conditions have been compared with those of healthy subjects who have been instructed to fake the symptom, such as not being able to move their left arm. The MRIs for the two groups are remarkably different. (While you don't need to be told your symptoms are real, this research is highlighting where possible treatments might be found.)

While orthodox[17] medicine is evolving around the world and adopting new research, medical treatment depends upon the cultural background of the practitioner.

Alternative or complementary medicine provides some interesting treatments but does not seek to meet the rigorous scientific standards of orthodox medicine. If it did, and was proven effective, it would be, by definition, included as orthodox.

---

17 The term 'orthodox' is preferred over the geographically nonsensical term 'Western medicine', because the principles of scientific method have been adopted worldwide now. To be accepted as orthodox, however, no longer means simply to be constrained to the narrow confines of the biomedical model. Plenty of evidence has proven that the biopsychosocial model is pertinent to the health outcomes of an individual. See chapter 8 for more on this model.

Chapter 7

The nocebo effect and the surprising influence of negative thoughts

We have all heard about the placebo effect. You may take an inert pill believing it is a potent medicine and go on to experience real benefit from the sham treatment. Or when a child hurts themselves and their mother kisses it better. Placebo. But what about the nocebo effect? And how might that be affecting – or hampering – your recovery? In this chapter, I explain all.

No morphine? No problem! The accidental discovery of placebo

Imagine a wounded soldier during World War II. The pain from his injuries is getting worse as the initial shock is wearing off. At last, he sees the medic, Dr Harry Beecher, coming and giving him a syringeful of morphine. He finally has relief from his terrible pain. He sinks into the opioid-induced state of calm and feels his pain seeping away. What he does not know is that, instead of the morphine he thought he had been given, he only received plain saline.

No analgesia at all. Earlier, Dr Beecher had found to his dismay that he had run out of morphine and yet the wounded soldiers kept on coming. With no option, he continued to inject them, replacing the morphine with saline solution. To his surprise, almost half the soldiers reported that the injection reduced or eased their pain.

So, how does placebo work?

How could a soldier with a war wound experience pain relief simply from saline? Researchers have now found that after you take a placebo, your brain releases endorphin, a morphine-like substance that modifies your pain experience – so long as you believe you have been given real analgesia. Further evidence that endorphins play a role in placebo is growing: if you take an opiate blocker, such as naloxone, at the same time as the placebo, the placebo does not work as well.

But this is not the whole story. Naloxone only partially blocks the painkilling properties of placebo. So, what else could be happening when you take a placebo?

Placebo can take many forms, not just a sugar pill. Injections, devices, even operations can have a placebo effect. Even a doctor who convinces that you will soon feel better is activating a placebo effect.

And it's not just pain that can benefit from placebo, either. Nearly any symptom may improve. Most properly conducted drug trials have a placebo group, where half the subjects are given a sham product. Even patients with Parkinson's disease may find their tremor is reduced when given a placebo pill. So, a placebo may be powerful and may help a lot of people, but doctors debate the ethics of using pills they know to be inert. Most conclude it is unethical to deceive and so avoid the use of placebo.

The complementary and alternate medicine market (defined here as the 'medicines' with no proven benefits beyond that expected from the placebo effect) accounts for $3.5 billion in expenditure each year in Australia and is used by two out of three people.

What are the possible reasons for this? One obvious reason is that the products truly have a pharmacologic effect beyond placebo, but no-one has done the testing.

But what are some of the other ways that these placebo products might work in the real world, other than through classical conditioning and the release of endorphin and dopamine?

Some conditions are simply self-limiting and would have got better anyway. Many people still believe that antibiotics are essential to recover from colds. However, no scientific evidence exists for antibiotics being effective against viral infections other than the placebo effect or the fact that the cold symptoms simply resolve during the taking of the pills.

Certain conditions such as multiple sclerosis or forms of arthritis have a natural cycle of flares and remission, the latter perhaps being misattributed to the taking of a placebo – that is, the recovery coincides with the natural remission in symptoms, rather than the effect of the sham medication.

Sometimes, when we find ourselves unwell, we change certain behaviours and start to take better care of ourselves – paying better attention, for example, to diet, exercise and rest. In other words, we activate the restorative and maintenance mode. The improved state of wellbeing can again be misattributed to the medication.

Taking a pill in the belief that it will cure you can also alter your perception of your symptoms – so, for example, the pain you were feeling is now interpreted as just an uncomfortable tingling. In other words, you stop paying attention to the pain and so notice it less.

With the expectation of a cure while taking the placebo, you can also have less anxiety, reducing adrenaline and hypervigilance in your system. And so you start to feel better.

An interesting brain phenomenon is also relevant here. This is 'remembered wellness', when the brain can respond to an imagined situation just like it was in the actual situation. This may have a role in how you respond when you take a placebo.

What else helps placebos to work?

A lot of characteristics of the placebo product can improve its effectiveness. Here are some of the more surprising research findings:

- A larger pill is more effective than a smaller pill, even with the same amount of drug (or placebo) contained.
- Taking two pills is more effective than taking one.
- Injections are more powerful than pills. Expensive procedures and surgery also have a strong placebo effect.
- Your attitude also matters. If you expect the treatment to work, the chances of a placebo effect are higher, but placebos can still work even if you are sceptical of success. The power of suggestion is at work here.
- The doctor–patient relationship has a role too. If you trust your healthcare practitioner, you are more likely to find that the placebo will work. When you have a strong relationship of trust with your medical providers, you release oxytocin, one of the many happiness hormones, and this blocks spinal cord neurons from sending pain signals to the brain.

Expectancy effect: The more you expect an effect, the more likely it will occur

As just mentioned, your attitude also matters, and this plays into the expectancy effect – that is, the more you expect a good result, the more likely the placebo will work. At the time of writing in Australia, doctors are amazed at the consumption of magnesium, which was shown years ago not to make any difference to symptoms such as muscle cramps or muscle aching or tiredness, when compared to placebo. And yet, people are reporting wonderful results from their nightly magnesium. A powerful placebo is working. Most doctors know that the supplements are unlikely to do harm and are safer than some alternatives, so are happy to keep quiet about the evidence and let the placebo work its magic.

Interestingly, some doctors take magnesium themselves, even though they know it is no better than placebo. But they also know that placebo is better than nothing, even when you know you are taking a dud.

A decade or so ago, everyone was taking another mineral, zinc, because it was believed to prevent infection, with slim evidence to back this up. Eventually most people stopped taking it. Expectations rise and fall quite mysteriously.

Can we do placebo-controlled experiments to prove the usefulness of every pill? Probably. For every operation? This is much more difficult and has been compared to doing a placebo-controlled test of whether parachutes work. Lack of volunteers may be a problem.

So, placebos have been and are used regularly. They bring benefit to patients, but are they entirely free of negative side effects? What happens if you believe you are taking a powerful medication with strong side effects? Can this medication cause harm, even if it is a placebo? Here we get to the nocebo effect.

The nocebo effect – the placebo effect's dark counterpart

> Sticks and stones will break your bones
> But words will never hurt you

You may have been told this as a child and, like me, believed it. But it turns out not to be true. The previous sections in this chapter outline how a placebo drug can have a beneficial effect on your body. But could a placebo drug create negative side effects? Could you experience what is called the nocebo effect? The nocebo effect is the evil twin of placebo. Instead of having a good response to a sugar pill, you suffer adverse effects. This, of course, is a functional symptom.

In her presentation 'This talk may cause side effects', from the 2022 Festival of Dangerous Ideas, nocebo effect expert Dr Kate Faasse related the following story:

> ### MR A AND THE POWER OF NEGATIVE THINKING
> A young man, Mr A, enrolled in a clinical trial for a new antidepressant medication. One day, after a huge fight with his girlfriend, Mr A took all the remaining 29 pills he'd been given for that study. Knowing he made a mistake, he got himself to hospital where he said, 'Help me, I took all my pills', before collapsing. The hospital staff raced into action. Mr A was drowsy, pale, sweating, breathing rapidly, and when they got him on monitoring equipment, it became clear that his heart rate was extremely high, and his blood pressure was very low. He was showing concerning signs of a drug overdose. When the physician from the clinical trial arrived, everyone expected to be told that Mr A had taken 29 antidepressant pills. What she revealed instead, was that he had taken 29 placebo pills, sugar pills, containing no active ingredient at all. So everyone in that room was relieved, but a little surprised at this information. But sure enough, within 15 minutes, Mr A was alert, sitting up, chatting to everyone in the room, and his blood pressure and heart rate had gone back to normal. So rather than a drug overdose, Mr A had taken a placebo [or nocebo] overdose.

Mr A obliged experts with an experiment about the power of the nocebo effect. Can it really be true that many symptoms we suffer are the result of this form of negative thinking? Can we truly make ourselves sick, if we simply believe the pill we have taken can do this?

The truth about the nocebo effect should have far-reaching effects on what we doctors tell our patients.

'Reading this may hurt you'

Dr Faasse has gone on to research what happens if you decide to read the consumer information for a new medication. Often a long list of possible adverse effects is provided. Is it possible that some of the reactions you might have are due to the nocebo effect? Of course, Dr Faasse has some elegantly designed trials to prove exactly that. In her studies, reported rates of adverse effects were recorded for two groups of patients: the first group was given a list of possible side effects; the second group was told nothing. You now might not be surprised to learn that the second group had much less in the way of side effects to report. As Dr Faasse outlined to me, 'We have created a vicious cycle, when we tell people a list of side effects that they could get. Some will then go ahead and develop those side effects. It is then reported that the drug definitely does create negative symptoms, and the story gets repeatedly reinforced.'

Statins cause muscle pain – or do they?

This is the sorry tale of the cholesterol-lowering drug group called statins. Although they have been proven to save lives, thousands of people across the world are putting their lives at risk by ceasing them, due to the belief that they are causing muscle pain. But are they the cause? To study this question, doctors rely on what is called the 'double blind, placebo-controlled trial', where neither the researchers nor the subjects know whether each coded pill is the drug or a harmless placebo. Only at the end of the trial is the code cracked and the results revealed.

A 2022 study published in medical journal *The Lancet*, involving over 100,000 people, showed that yes, 27.1 per cent of people taking the statin developed muscle pain or weakness. But here's the critical issue: so did 26.6 per cent of the people taking the placebo! Researchers describe the 'absolute excess risk' of experiencing muscle symptoms in the first year in the group taking statins as equivalent to 11 per 1000 patients, but the vast majority are suffering from the nocebo effect.[18]

---

18 For full details of this study, see 'Effect of statin therapy on muscle symptoms: An individual participant data meta-analysis of large-scale, randomised, double-blind trials', *The Lancet*, 29 August 2022, www.thelancet.com/journals/lancet/article/PIIS0140-6736(22)01545-8/fulltext#%20.

Sadly, for the statin class of drug, doctors are largely failing to change the discourse. The power of nocebo surpasses the power of science and reason.

Nocebo effects are classic functional symptoms. Their cause is not physical, but a complex interplay of societal and psychological factors. But not everyone suffers from the nocebo effect. Here the science is once again helpful in showing why.

What makes you more likely to suffer from a nocebo effect?

Negative expectations from a consultation with your doctor are more likely to result in a poor outcome. If you have a fundamental mistrust of the doctor, the treatment or the procedure you are having, you are more likely to have a poor response to treatment.

The COVID vaccinations caused a lot of illness, with much higher levels of adverse effects than are usual with vaccines. It is not possible to prove how many of these reactions were due to physical side effects and how much was the nocebo effect.[19]

The importance of a healthy, trusting relationship is so important for your health.

'Informed' consent

In modern times, you can expect to be given sufficient information about any pills or procedures your healthcare team is advising, and their potential side effects, before deciding whether to accept it. However, what if the warnings about the potential complications or side effects of the treatment result in you experiencing a nocebo effect? If you are told the pill might cause nausea or headache, is

---

19 JAMA Netw Open. 2023 Mar; 6(3): e234732. Published online 2023 Mar 27. doi: 10.1001/jamanetworkopen.2023.4732. PMCID: PMC10043751. PMID: 36972051. Expectations and Prior Experiences Associated With Adverse Effects of COVID-19 Vaccination.

it possible for you to develop these symptoms simply as a result of conditioning?

From an ethical position, is it right for your doctor to carefully inform you of every possible risk, no matter how unlikely, but, as a result, you decide against treatment, which is likely to lead to a worse outcome?

> Although informed consent requires you be given the list of possible adverse reactions, such information can serve you poorly.

Often, informed consent is given in this manner:

Doctor: *So, you have been diagnosed with Z syndrome. I recommend you take X.*

Patient: *What are the side effects of X?*

Doctor: *Well, here is the list – headaches, nausea, rashes.*

Patient: *Maybe I will just try my luck with what my naturopath gives me. Her treatments don't have any side effects.*

What is usually not included in the discussion is the obvious risk of leaving your condition untreated.

So, the pernicious effect of nocebo symptoms can have very real consequences. Functional symptoms have many unfortunate consequences and it is time that we all take a good hard look at them and their role in our health choices.

What can you do to avoid suffering from the nocebo effect?

You and your doctor can work to reduce the likelihood of you having adverse outcomes from the nocebo effect in a few different ways:

- When any new treatment is discussed, it is important that the likely benefit is discussed with less emphasis on the possible negative effects. In other words, usually the doctor can reassure you that they would themselves accept the treatment, knowing the relative risks of treating versus not treating.
- Make sure you get clear information about what to do if a problem with the treatment emerges – this 'safety netting' can help mitigate concern and hence reduce the risk.
- Good reliable sources of information about your condition and the best treatment can help support your choice to commit to the treatment with less concern. Less anxiety about having treatment will reduce your stress-related symptoms and make the treatment more tolerable.
- Make sure you have a clear understanding of how to take your treatment and what is reasonable to expect. The focus should be on the likely benefits, rather than the unlikely risks. After all, your doctor has a genuine commitment to improving your health and a strong ethical commitment to (we say it in Latin, for emphasis) *primum non nocere*; first, do no harm.

To summarise this chapter, one reason functional symptoms can occur is due to the nocebo effect. These are genuine symptoms, but not due to a physical disease. Dr Faasse has proven that simply being told about side effects makes them more likely.

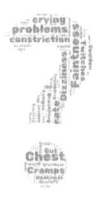

Chapter 8

Why the biomedical system is failing you – and where to turn to now

In the present day, we are in the thrall of science and technology – and for good reason.

The history of medicine is an extraordinary journey from superstition and innumerable unsubstantiated theories about health and disease to today's strong emphasis on evidence-based diagnosis and treatment. This has been a truly wonderful development, where accurate diagnosis of disease is followed by proven treatments. This 'biomedical model' has come not only to dominate the working framework of most doctors but may also have come to affect your own understanding of the cause of illness, and how it is diagnosed and treated.

The more a doctor is welded onto the biomedical paradigm – that is, 'if it can't be measured, it doesn't exist' – the more your functional symptoms will drive them to despair. And vice versa: the more you believe there must be a test to find the physical disease that explains your symptoms, the more frustrating will be your efforts (presuming your doctor has already done adequate examinations and investigations).

So, if you have symptoms that don't fit into the narrow confines of this biomedical paradigm, you may find yourself relegated to the fringes, often having to fend for yourself, and further burdened with the suspicion that you may be thought of as fake, a malingerer or a 'stress case'.

But it doesn't have to be that way.

Disease versus illness

Throughout the history of medicine, functional symptoms have had various explanations that satisfied both healer and patient. Whether it was an imbalance in energies or an ill wind or a curse, a socially acceptable means of explaining what was happening would be agreed upon.

But while the biomedical model is excellent at diagnosing physical disease, it cannot define, let alone heal, any condition that has unique manifestations and normal tests. The strict criteria needed to be met for a condition to be diagnosed means that biomedical conditions need to be the same in everybody.

Beyond reductionism

The biomedical model relies on the reductionist approach – that is, the belief that human behaviour, including illness, can be explained by breaking it down into smaller component parts.

Using the reductionist approach, the modern doctor will gather similar cases, identify the shared physiological disturbances, describe the usual natural history of the disease and define the best treatment. For example, when pneumonia arises, a patient will typically have shortness of breath, cough and fever. Blood tests show increased white cells and a chest X-ray reveals changes in a well-defined pattern. If the diagnosis is not clear, the doctor will do more and more sensitive tests until the abnormal part is identified.

But understanding the nature of a functional disorder requires the doctor to put aside this reductionist approach and be willing to explore the causation of symptoms unique to this patient's experience.

When all your tests are normal, and yet you are unwell, we need to move away from the orthodox realm of biomedicine and towards a broader understanding of health. Fortunately, we have made a lot of progress here.

George Engel and the biopsychosocial model

In 1977, American psychiatrist George Engel proposed a model of health and disease to challenge the standard biomedical model. This model – the biopsychosocial model – asserts that illness is a result of many factors. Health experts are still grappling with the concepts nearly 50 years on.

The following figure highlights the elements that make up Engel's biopsychosocial model.

George Engel's biopsychosocial model

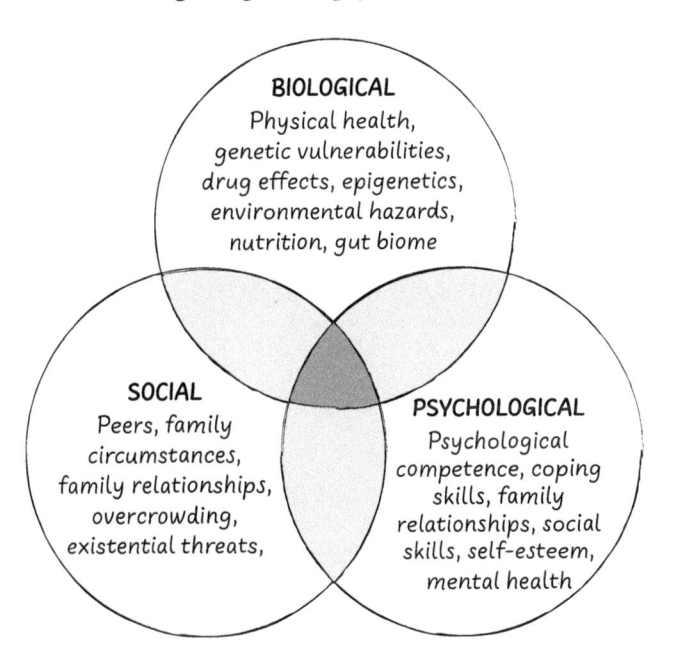

BIOLOGICAL
Physical health, genetic vulnerabilities, drug effects, epigenetics, environmental hazards, nutrition, gut biome

SOCIAL
Peers, family circumstances, family relationships, overcrowding, existential threats,

PSYCHOLOGICAL
Psychological competence, coping skills, family relationships, social skills, self-esteem, mental health

While the elements included in Engel's model may seem obvious to some, these factors are not often included in the standard history-taking of doctors even today. The normal expectation about what happens in an encounter with your doctor is that the doctor will seek to elicit the reason for your visit. You are likely to describe your symptoms. The doctor will seek more information about your symptoms. In Australia, GPs are trained to enquire into the biopsychosocial, and also now sexual, context that was present when your symptom arose, but in the increasing haste of modern consultations, this may be overlooked, especially if the biomedical model is dominant.

Listening for a few minutes to symptoms and then ordering investigations of the affected region is poor medicine. Inexperienced doctors may rely on tests more than their clinical judgement. (Such reliance also brings in the risk of 'false positives'.)[20] Such shoddy treatment is likely to send you down the wrong path.

But if you are fortunate enough to be seeing a doctor who is familiar with you and your family's health and circumstances, and can consider all the factors Engel outlined that may affect your health, you are a long way towards having your health problem understood in a broader framework.

> If your doctor can incorporate your cultural influences, belief systems and sexual issues into what is causing the illness, they can begin to bring a better understanding.

Aaron's story is an example of this.

---

20 A 'false positive' is when the test results suggest you have the disease being tested for, but you don't. Most tests have a percentage of false positives. Your doctor should be aware of this risk and should ensure the test is done only if the result will make sense, given your presentation.

AARON

Aaron rarely needed to see me because he kept in good shape and was blessed with a strong constitution, so when he started to attend frequently with headaches, I knew something was up. A full examination and brain scans revealed nothing more than muscle tension. And yet, the headaches persisted. Eventually, I was able to get the story: Aaron was happily married with three lovely children, but to his horror, he had fallen in love with his wife's best friend's husband. An obsessive love affair had started. Deeply unhappy, he eventually shared the truth with his wife. They worked through the issue together – the affair ended and so did the headaches.

Aaron was able to reflect on the huge strains that his affair had created and that he needed to resolve, which included his valued relationships, his love of his family, his home, his social interactions, his sexual identity and his view of himself as an honest man. In the light of this, it was not surprising that he got a few headaches.

Dr Engel's construct helps us to appreciate the role that life plays in our health. But we need more than this. We need a systematic means to understand your symptoms, exclude risk of disease and develop a way forward.

We can use the flag system to organise our thinking.

Flags: Red, yellow and green

Flags are one of the methods used by doctors to sort out whether or not your symptoms could be due to a physical cause that needs to be treated. They also help to focus our attention on what else should be done.

Red flags

For every condition, doctors learn a list of 'red flags' to look out for because these suggest the possibility of more serious disease.

Red flags are symptoms, signs or history that indicate possible serious pathology and, hence, support the decision to investigate further. If no red flags are present, the risk of serious pathology is negligible, and the patient can be reassured that further testing is not needed and they can be treated with conservative measures.

Red flags for lower back pain, for example, include:

- recent significant trauma
- (prolonged or systemic) glucocorticoid use
- osteoporosis
- age younger than 20 or older than 55 years
- radiculopathy (pain radiating down a leg)
- bladder or bowel dysfunction
- severe or progressive sensory or motor disturbance
- history of malignancy
- unexplained weight loss
- pain worse at night or at rest
- fever/chills/fatigue
- immune compromise
- intravenous drug use
- history of inflammatory arthritis, enthesitis or uveitis
- morning stiffness or improvement with movement.

Red flags are what doctors should ask you about because they are associated with a higher likelihood that your symptoms may be due to a serious physical condition and should prompt further testing.

The exclusion of red flags is essential and helps to suggest that your symptoms are not likely to be serious.

If no sign of physical disease is detected, then it is usual for your doctor to offer treatment for your symptoms, such as pain relief or some rest from work, to allow time for your body to recover. The opportunity to be reviewed within a reasonable time should be agreed upon.

So, for the majority of functional symptoms, the treatment is based on:
- education and reassurance
- perhaps some symptom relief
- agreed time for review.

For most functional symptoms, this approach is effective. But persistent or troubling symptoms need careful consideration. Your doctor will need to explore all possible factors.

Yellow flags

Asking about the presence of 'yellow flags' can help your doctor to identify what *might* contribute to your symptoms and possible treatment plans.

Yellow flags are psychosocial factors that increase the risk that your functional condition could result in long-term disability and potential loss of work.

Yellow flags include:
- fear and consequent avoidance behaviour
- a belief that pain and activity are harmful or severely disabling
- sickness behaviours
- low mood, anxiety
- social withdrawal
- the expectation that passive treatment rather than active participation will help
- issues with the compensation system
- poor job satisfaction or work-related stress
- overprotective family
- lack of social support, loneliness, despondency
- financial problems
- somaticising tendency – the tendency to express your emotions in physical form
- frequent or persisting symptoms

- multiple symptoms
- tendency to catastrophise (thinking the worst)
- feelings of helplessness/hopelessness, health-related anxiety
- passive, overactive or suppressive behaviour (for example, protective and avoidance behaviour, persistent industriousness/perseverance, safety-seeking behaviour)
- addiction
- PTSD.

If you have any of the yellow flags just listed, revealing them to your doctor can be helpful. These problems can then be addressed, and doing so may expedite your recovery.

Who would have thought that poor job satisfaction or an overprotective family could increase your likelihood of ongoing functional symptoms? But this has been found to be true in study after study. The trouble is, when you are the one with the pain, it is very hard to recognise this pattern. In chapter 14, I explore some of the means that might help you recognise the patterns and respond to them in a constructive fashion.

However, an overly simplistic psychosocial explanation can be disempowering. It creates a victimisation and further reinforces a passive role whereby the sufferer remains at the mercy of social forces beyond their control. This is particularly the case for those situations where there are neither the words to express a problem nor the power to disregard societal pressures. Children are very prone to this. Another vulnerable group are those who have had a family member suffer from a delayed diagnosis.

Finally, the list provided in chapter 3 of the causes of functional conditions included genetics and epigenetics, which may explain why you and not your co-workers have symptoms in the same work situation. But as you cannot usually identify genetic causes or do anything about these factors, they rarely are mentioned, but almost certainly have a role in every functional condition.

So, what if the cause of your symptom cannot be found?

It is not uncommon for a functional condition to be diagnosed without a cause being found. The many trivial glitches we all experience, such as a hiccup or eye-twitch, are rarely due to a known cause. Similarly, more serious or long-lasting symptoms can also occur without an obvious reason.

Your doctor may run through questions to try to determine whether certain factors may be contributing to your condition. This is like asking a heart attack survivor if they smoke. It is important to identify risk factors because they can affect the outcome: ongoing smoking increases the risk of further heart disease. But once they have been ruled out, your focus can safely turn to treatment trials.

> Unlike physical disease, the treatment of functional conditions can proceed without agreement on the cause.

Once your functional symptom has been diagnosed, it can help to identify your strengths and turn your attention towards developing them. These protective factors are called 'green flags'.

Green flags

Green flags are the qualities associated with a likelihood of a good and timely recovery from your functional symptoms. They are protective factors, and include the following:

- a healthy outlook – for example, self-confidence and good sense of humour
- active coping strategies that increase your chances of a favourable outcome – for example, participation in sports, ability to enjoy yourself and relax
- your personal resources, such as hobbies, general motivation and job-related plans

- no or minimal pressures at home or work – for example, good social support and satisfactory workplace
- no mental illness
- your ability to continue functioning normally despite your symptoms.

So, where to from here?

Once you have accepted that your symptoms are functional and have a good understanding of what may have contributed to their development (if anything), you need to turn your focus towards what can be done to facilitate your recovery.

Your doctor may have done a battery of tests, and you may be waiting for further specialist investigations to be certain no physical cause is present. I would encourage you to undertake the path outlined in the following chapters, while you wait for your specialist appointment. It will do no harm and may help.

In the chapters so far, we've explored a lot of information about how functional conditions can arise. To help deepen your understanding, I now give you Maree's story, written in her own words.[21] I then identify the factors that triggered her body entering into defensive mode.

Maree's journey is revealing, both in how serious functional conditions can be and in how they can arise in wonderfully active, hardworking people.

MAREE TELLS HER STORY OF GOING TO HELL AND BACK

Six years ago after the birth of my second child, I had a retained placenta, lost quite a lot of blood, I needed to go under general anaesthetic to remove the placenta and stitch the rupture in my cervix. I was given a blood transfusion and iron tablets. After this point, I also started putting lots of pressure on myself to

---

21 Maree is not my patient.

start my master's degree and plan our wedding (scheduled for four months after my son was born). I was having periods of feeling generally unwell (fatigue, nausea, vertigo) that would come and go. I went to the doctors, but they said my bloods were all fine so no issue.

After the wedding I had an episode of body tremors and generally very fatigued, feeling anxious and depressed. I went to a counsellor who helped, and I started to feel like I was getting my energy and motivation back when I fell pregnant again. (My copper coil had fallen out without me realising!)

My third pregnancy was difficult with fatigue, nausea and catching every bug going. I was worried I was going to be sick for the birth, but my body cleverly bounced back to give birth, and all went fine. I felt a boost of energy after that and started doing four spin classes a week and booked a family holiday to Spain when my daughter was 12 weeks old. A week after getting back, I hit a very bad period of fatigue, aches and nausea ... I actually became very paranoid and anxious that I was pregnant again, even though the pregnancy tests were negative, and I paid for a private scan to make sure. I went to the doctors again who diagnosed me with Gilbert syndrome,[22] but said it was totally harmless so nothing to do with my symptoms.

I kept trying to push through to get my energy back, and that's when I also started the aerial silks. When my daughter was four months, I performed in an aerial Christmas show and even though I felt awful I kept pushing on. I then got a virus (pretty sure it was COVID because it was just spreading around that time) which really floored me. Fortunately, everything was locked down and I was forced to stop and recover. Even then, I was only getting four to six hours of sleep, trying to juggle everything.

I was starting to feel better but once lockdown rules eased, I went back into pushing myself to finish my master's degree and build my business more and take on more complex behaviour cases and earn more money. I had another bout of illness and COVID over the following Christmas and then decided to start working with a business coach to expand. Even

---

22 Gilbert syndrome is a common liver condition that is considered harmless, with no treatment recommended.

at this point I was feeling very burnt out, but I kept pushing forward because it was 'what should be done'. There was a voice inside telling me not to do it and that I wasn't enjoying the work anymore, but I had just spent all that time and money doing my master's to become a clinical animal behaviourist so I had to keep going – otherwise, I would be a total failure. My anxiety, fatigue, tremors, brain fog and body pains were getting worse, and I couldn't keep up with all the demands from work and being a parent. I would then beat myself up about not being good enough and keep pushing on.

Then one night I had a three-hour episode of full body tremors. I had to stay in bed for a few days, but I did slowly get back up and do more with help but now I had this awful constant sense of dread, fatigue and anxiety about things getting worse. In the past when I had experienced the periods of fatigue, I was always worried it would stay but they usually went away after a while. However, this time it wasn't going away.

The doctors prescribed me beta blockers so I would take one to help my nerves about work but after three days of taking them I was even worse. I went to a job and had to leave early. I felt totally disoriented, spaced out and panicky, and had bad stomach pains.

It was then the Easter holidays, and both my parents and husband were going to be away so I would be looking after the kids myself. I didn't want to ask for help or ruin anyone else's plans and I was so desperate for things to just go back to normal that I told my parents and Damien to go and not worry about me.

Over that week I could feel my mind and body starting to break but I kept going, and then on the Friday evening my body started to feel very weird, and I had a panic attack. I had another panic attack that night and took more beta blockers. I truly thought I was going to die, and my poor kids would find my body with no-one there to look after them. My mum came back from holiday the next day to help, and I kept taking the beta blockers, but things got much worse, and I had a week of almost constant panic attacks to the point where I couldn't even spend a minute by myself in the house or with the kids. The furthest

I could walk was to the bottom of the lane outside our house without my body going into overload and shutting down.

After this point I was at my very worst and couldn't do much without having to go and lie down again. It felt like my nervous system was a faulty car alarm and just setting off all the time over nothing. My sleep was very badly affected, I had pain in my joints and body, and I kept getting migraines and tension headaches. I was so scared that I wouldn't be able to look after my kids again and be the mum that I had so enjoyed being. I was also angry with myself for pushing so much with work when that now seemed totally meaningless in my current situation. I got back in touch with the doctor but the only option they had for me was to take anti-anxiety medication, and after my experience with the beta blockers I had a huge fear about taking anything else.

Maree's journey to recovery is continued in chapter 13.

Maree had no red flags, some yellow flags and plenty of green flags, so although she had work to do, she was likely to recover.

Like Maree, most patients with persistent fatigue battle for months before recovery can occur, albeit slowly. We know that persistent fatigue is probably a multifactorial condition, so we need to keep an open mind about all possibilities.

The figure overleaf provides a forensic analysis of Maree's story, outlining the predisposing and precipitating factors, and the consequent symptoms.

The predisposing and precipitating factors behind Maree's symptoms

PREDISPOSING FACTORS	PRECIPITATING FACTORS	SYMPTOMS
Two pregnancies – stress on the body Lots of pressure on self: Two babies + study + wedding Ongoing pressure to overachieve	Severe blood loss Sleep loss Wedding stress Third pregnancy too soon Competitive sports (silks) Overworking COVID Money stress Sleep disturbance	Fatigue Nausea Vertigo Tremors Anxiety Depression Recurrent infections Worry Aches Unwell Exhaustion Brain fog Panic attacks Physical weakness Sleep disturbance

Now let's take a look at her symptoms within the body stress systems:

1. *Autonomic nervous system:*
   - blood loss/anaemia (leads to increased heart rate and other stress responses)
   - excessive workload: study/work/business/family.
2. *Hormone system:*
   - multiple pregnancies with inadequate recovery
   - obstetric complications.

3. *Immune-inflammatory system:*
   - recurrent viral illnesses.
4. *Circadian rhythm:*
   - sleep quality and quantity disrupted.
5. *Skeletomotor system:*
   - physically demanding activities beyond natural capacity.
6. *Microbiome–gut–brain system:*
   - suboptimal nutrition.
7. *Brain system:*
   - mental demands with excessive work and business pressures
   - personality vulnerabilities – response to perceived underachievement is to push harder
   - self-criticism and anger towards self
   - underlying anxiety.

Is it any wonder Maree's system broke down? Maree's journey to recovery is included in chapter 13 to illustrate how recovery can be possible.

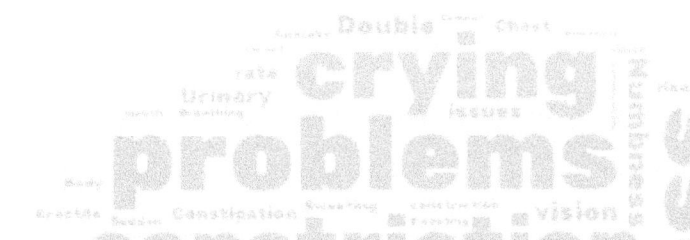

Part III: The path to recovery

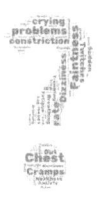

Chapter 9

Step 1: Get a clear diagnosis

As outlined so far in this book, functional conditions are complex, with multiple causes, some of which are inherited or untreatable. The rest of this book focuses on what you and your healthcare team can do to alleviate your symptoms.

This might be a good time to have a notebook to capture the insights that you find helpful. Share your thoughts with your support team and build a plan for your recovery.

If you are dealing with a functional condition, you know that it is quite difficult to get a clear diagnosis. Given everything discussed in the earlier chapters, you may now see why your functional condition is tricky to diagnose. It is even more difficult to explain. While having a functional condition is extremely common, your expressed symptoms are unique, so there is no simple way to label your condition.

It can co-exist with an existing physical illness, but just be worse. For example, you may have proven asthma, but then find yourself more breathless. Is this an exacerbation of the asthma or a functional breathing problem?

You may also find that your symptoms can shift and drift around your body in a most exasperating way. Just when you have had your headaches thoroughly investigated, you may find you have developed an upset gut or debilitating fatigue, and the cycle of medical investigations and, if the cause is functional, frustrating lack of answers ensues. You feel you are getting nowhere.

Here, we are going to take a radical approach to explain the cause of your symptoms and their treatment, but this needs you to really understand the reasoning.

A risk factor is not the cause

Doctors experienced in treating functional conditions can identify risk factors for developing a functional disorder, just like a cardiologist might find risk factors for heart disease. However, the fact that risk factors exist does not mean a heart attack is going to happen. It is just more likely in smokers than non-smokers. Similarly, if someone has had a heart attack, it would be stupid to assume that they have smoked.

In the case of functional conditions, the same holds true. Just because certain factors have been shown to be associated with functional conditions does not mean that they must be present in every person with a functional condition. For example, many people who have a traumatic childhood do not go on to develop functional symptoms, but such symptoms are more likely in those with a traumatic past. And not everyone with a functional condition has had a traumatic past.

Focusing on a diagnosis

We need to assume that you have symptoms, and that you have been to at least one doctor who has completed a thorough medical history, examination and appropriate investigations to exclude any physical causes. You first need to give a careful account of your symptoms to your doctor, who would be holding several ideas about your possible diagnosis in their head and would ask questions to rule out any red flags (refer to the previous chapter) or physical diagnoses. They would then give you a physical examination to check for signs of changes in your body. Certain tests may be done but your doctor should be able to reassure you of the likelihood of the functional nature of your problem, even while doing tests to make sure that any possible physical condition is excluded.

Once these physical conditions have been excluded, the next step is to determine what functional condition(s) you have. This is essential. A clear diagnosis is what leads to a clear treatment plan. Your diagnosis may also include a discussion of the three categories of functional disorders: persistent functional symptoms, functional somatic syndromes and somatic stress disorders (refer to chapter 2).

By now, it should be clear that everyone has the occasional functional symptom, but for some, these are more troublesome and need a plan of treatment. You may have several functional conditions from all three categories, in which case you would need a multidisciplinary team to help evolve a management plan to aid your recovery.

Unfortunately, often the understanding that your symptom is most likely functional is withheld from you. This is not helpful and can lead to unnecessary worry. Again, about one in three symptoms seen by your doctor has the likelihood of being functional. Testing is often ordered, not because your doctor is worried necessarily that there is something physical but simply to reassure you that they are taking the symptom seriously.

Medical studies into the value of testing shows that a vast number of tests are unnecessary and wasteful, but the 'lawyer in the room', patient expectation and perhaps a lack of confidence in the doctor about their diagnosis can all lead to excessive testing.

Regardless of testing or not, you should be given a clear explanation of why your condition most likely does not fulfil the criteria of a physical condition. This is usually obvious to doctors.

DIAGNOSIS: DON'T TRY THIS AT HOME

Doctors train for years for a reason: diagnosis is difficult, even in the best hands. Your best chance of getting the right diagnosis is to give a clear account of *all* your symptoms in an orderly fashion. Ideally, your doctor knows your past health conditions, because this is important information, so make sure your records are up to date. Remember – while you are the expert of your experience, your doctor holds the expertise of diagnosing. Work together until you reach agreement.

While it is tempting to surf the net to find out what is wrong with you, this may not be in your best interest. For one thing, to be able to return to your restorative mode, you need time to eat healthily, be active, optimise your mental health, engage socially and sleep. Ask yourself if you are able to do these essential activities while spending hours on your computer.

Another reason is that most websites focus on the physical diseases, so if you search something like, 'I am having chest pain', the sites will immediately mention heart attack or pneumonia. Of course, that is what your doctor will be thinking to exclude as soon as they see you, but if you walk in looking worried but otherwise well, and your physical examination and office tests are normal, then your doctor can often rapidly reassure you, even if further tests are being done to be sure it is nothing serious. But if you are talking only to 'Dr Google', you could worry yourself sick in no time.

Of course, once you have been given a diagnosis by your doctor, the internet can be very helpful to provide a full explanation of your conditions and all the things you might do to help you recover.

Once you and your doctor agree that your symptom is likely to be functional, the next step is to get beyond the symptom and consider the cause – covered in the next chapter.

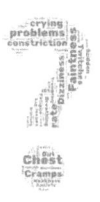

Chapter 10

Step 2: Shift the focus from treating the symptom to treating the cause

Focusing less on your symptoms and more on their cause may surprise you, because this is the very opposite to the usual approach to symptoms. But, given all that you read about in the earlier chapters, two things must now be obvious:

1. Your functional symptoms may have arisen from a disturbance in the usual regulation of your body stress systems.
2. Unlike purely physical conditions, functional symptoms get worse the more you focus on them.

This is a new medical paradigm – that is, functional conditions are fundamentally different from ordinary physical symptoms, with a different causation and effect on your health. This means you need a different way to engage with your treating team. If you have read this far, it is likely that you have tried standard means to cure your symptoms and that has not worked. Why not explore some alternatives?

Quietening your internal body stress systems

Taking the following two steps towards your recovery is crucial:

1. *You need to turn your focus **away** from your symptoms:* The most positive approach, if possible, is simply to get on with your life, while arranging a timely review with your doctor. If you think back, you may recall previous weird symptoms that came and went mysteriously. Many of the patients presenting to their doctor with a functional symptom have found this simple measure is all that is required. This doesn't always work, however – in which case, the next step is also required.

2. *You need to turn your attention **towards** the quietening and regulating of your internal body stress systems:* As covered in chapters 3 and 4, an activated defensive mode can disrupt your body's normal functioning. So the importance of taking any stressors off your body systems and regaining and maintaining the restorative mode should be your priority.

This is easy to say but difficult to do. The rest of the book will focus on how to achieve this.

Using a simple example of functional back pain, once your doctor has ruled out red flags and identified the pain as likely to be related to your lifestyle, addressing the following possible causes can help:

- Is poor posture contributing to your pain?
- How many hours do you remain in one position?
- How often throughout the day do you move your back through its full range of movement?
- How much tension is in your life that tightens your muscles?
- How strong are your core muscles to assist with back support?
- Is the quality of your sleep inadequate to allow healing?

Doctors with a full waiting room may not have the time to help you identify all these factors and might simply prescribe you an analgesic, which won't really resolve your problem. And if you are inclined to worry that your pain could be a harbinger of something more serious, you can begin to enter the vicious cycle of triggering a greater body stress system activation and your pain could take over your life – a terrible outcome when the symptom rather than the causes is focused upon.

Addressing your doubts

You may have read and accepted all the previous chapters, but still believe that your symptoms must have a physical cause. I have several patients whom I have failed to convince otherwise and I can sum up their reasons:

- *'My symptom is so severe, it can't be functional.'* Doctors who specialise in functional conditions know that their patients often have worse pain, more disability and a poorer response to medical treatment than those with physical conditions. For example, patients with epilepsy generally have seizures that are shorter and easier to control than those with functional seizures (proven by EEG). As mentioned in chapter 5, functional pain is often more severe and disabling.
- *'It's not functional, because I took treatment x [such as antibiotics] and I got better … for a while.'* Most people underestimate the power of placebo. Functional symptoms fluctuate in an unpredictable fashion and any means of returning to the restorative mode will help. The comfort of being given definitive treatment is a potent placebo for some.
- *'I have adapted to my condition/disability and see no need to change.'* This is rarely said so explicitly, but sometimes when increased family support, NDIS and other forms of compensation are in place, some patients prefer to live with their symptoms because of the compensatory benefits such as a steady income, support services and other benefits they lacked before their symptoms developed. The yellow flags help to identify the well-documented barriers to recovery.

Modes and systems

From now on, for you to truly understand the new paradigm, you need to view your symptoms through the prism of modes and systems.

Remember – your health relies on your body remaining in the restorative and maintenance mode for most of the time in order to repair and rejuvenate itself. The defensive mode should be utilised during the situations that threaten your body, and then you need to ensure you return to your restorative mode.

> For mental and physical wellbeing, you need to spend most of your time in restorative mode.

We will also need to know which of your seven body stress systems, as outlined in chapter 4, have been disrupted.

If your symptoms persist even while you are trying to shift your focus *away* from them, it is time for a deeper understanding of your problem.

This step, the shift of focus from symptom to cause, is vital but is the exact opposite of usual treatment, so you need to really understand the reasoning here.

Note: While it helps to know what has activated our body stress system, sometimes no cause can be identified. In this case, you must skip this step and simply go straight to step 3 (outlined in the next chapter).

Are you in defensive mode now?

Remember that the cause of your functional symptom is the activation of your body stress systems, which occurs when your defensive mode is triggered. So, it is essential to be able to recognise when you are in your defensive mode and how often throughout the day and night you are activating it. This, of course, includes when your symptoms are active, but also when you have any other symptom related to an upregulated mode. See the list provided in chapter 2 for clues. For example, you may be tolerating such things as a rapid heart rate without acknowledging your body stress activation.

Many of the defensive mode responses are subconscious – you may not be aware of the hunching of your shoulders, for example, or your disturbed breathing or gut churning while you are fixated on your problems. I have patients who rely on worn devices to notify them, but it is better to take time out of your day to reset your restorative mode, such as by a session of meditation or a relaxing swim followed by a rest. Observe how your body feels and note how you might 'gear up' as you enter the busy time of day when you need to meet various demands. Many people do not realise that the resetting of their restorative mode is meant to serve as a reminder of how they need to be throughout much of the day. This will require practice, sometimes over months, to achieve. But it will make all the difference to your condition.

This may be sounding like just one more pressure on you. And you might feel guilty or a failure that you cannot maintain your restorative mode. It is important that you get a lot of support during this time to celebrate your steps to recovery and to keep going when you feel you have not made the progress you expect. Many people living with functional conditions have the habit of 'pushing through' to achieve their goals. The advice now is to do the exact opposite, and this can be challenging.

> Remember that our prime goal is to achieve the establishment of your restorative mode, so that you can repair any damage and remove debris that is essential for healthy body and brain functioning. Also, it will facilitate the return to normal working of your systems so your functional symptoms can abate.

Moving to the restorative mode

Think of that time when you were totally at ease without a worry in the world, relaxed and free. Let's call this a zero. Now picture a time when you were stressed out of your wits. That's a 10. Now, ask yourself where on the line between zero and 10 you spend most of your day. Do you wake up and enjoy the morning peace and spend some time in quiet contemplation (zero to one) or do you immediately gear up, rushing to get out of the house on time (five or six)? How are you during mundane activities like commuting? Are you calmly making your way through the world or is there always some pressure on your mind? Go right through your day, taking note of your internal state, right up to bedtime, and check if you prepare for a deep, restorative sleep. Or are you still in your defensive mode, meaning your sleep will be poor, your vital circadian rhythm disrupted and your main opportunity to heal missed?

Keeping an open – and inquiring – mind

Because it may have taken you a long time to be correctly diagnosed, many symptoms may have become 'hardwired' into your body stress systems and can take a considerable effort to modify. But, like Carmen and Vero from chapter 2, this modification is possible.

Of course, the experts on functional conditions, such as Dr Kozlowska, utilise several treatments to aid recovery, from physiotherapists to occupational therapists and psychologists who specialise in this area. I strongly recommend that you seek these experts out.

But if these experts are not available, finding a way forward requires you to seek out and be bold enough to try ... anything! A scientific criticism of alternative therapy is that many of them are 'unproven'. This is true in that any treatment of your unique condition cannot be tested in a double-blind placebo-controlled trial. So, you are left in the invidious position of being denied a medical diagnosis, and therefore a tested medical treatment.

You have a condition that medical science cannot measure (except with exceptional tools such as a functional MRI, which do show changes and where exciting new research is taking place). So, once you feel confident that your tests are normal, and medical science has little to offer you, it is sensible to seek any means that helps to return you to your natural restorative mode.

Luckily, science can still be used to test these therapies – but you need to be both the scientist and the subject. Take a note of how your symptoms are prior to engaging in any therapy. It is best to be quite rigorous in this: write down the level of your pain or severity of your symptom prior to treatment. Then try to fully engage without any reservation in whatever treatment you are willing to try. Only after the therapy, be sure to coolly evaluate your response. (Researchers call these experiments 'N=1'. The number of subjects being studied is one.) Check with your therapist when you could reasonably expect to see changes.

The usual cautions need to be heeded:

- Do not pay more than you can afford – doing so will create a further stressor.
- Ensure that your healthcare team, even if that is one doctor, is aware of your trial.
- Report back what the results were – this is science.

A cynic may suggest that these alternative therapies utilise only the placebo effect. Even if this is true, so long as you gain benefit, this is safe and effective. Go ahead! The proof of effective therapy is your recovery.

Throughout this book, I have used the terms 'defensive' and 'restorative' modes. However, these are not commonly used and you will find many other terms that approximate them. Traditional Chinese medicine refers to an imbalance in your 'qi'. Modern-day therapists talk about things like 'polyvagal theory'. Whatever modality you use, the purpose is to restore your body stress systems to normal.

How do you know if you are on the right track? Your symptoms will tell you. But it is important not to fixate on occasional setbacks or bad days. Maree (from chapter 8 and more in chapter 13) has a wonderful expression: *float through the dips*, meaning that you accept that setbacks will occur (and you may have no explanation for them) but don't judge or blame yourself. Simply, be kind to yourself and wait for the dip to pass, and then return to your plan for recovery.

You need to play the long game and be charting your recovery over weeks to months. Patience and perseverance is essential. Get support from family and friends and keep going. Seek out others with your condition and join supportive groups.

One proviso about groups: ensure they are focused on the journey to recovery, rather than the condition itself. An unhealthy dynamic can form when a group of people bond closely over shared symptoms. If one person starts to recover and pulls away, the rest of the group ideally celebrates this. If you find that the opposite happens, get out of that group – or you may be ill for a very long time.

To summarise step 2:
- Turn your focus from your symptom.
- Focus on remaining in restorative and maintenance mode.
- Utilise any therapy that enables this.

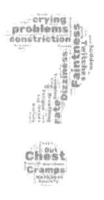

Chapter 11

Step 3: Identify which of your body stress systems are activated

Assuming you have identified how often your defensive mode is activated (refer to the previous chapter), the next step is to clarify which of your seven body stress systems have been upregulated, to choose the best means to reset them to the restorative mode.

For example, if your skeletomotor system is your predominant problem – with, say, aches and pains and muscle tension – you might choose to focus on the various physical means to recover, such as regular gentle exercise, massage, swimming, tai chi, yoga and physiotherapy.

Whereas, if it is your microbiome–gut–brain system that is disrupted and you have bowel upset and pains, you might choose to focus on what, how and when, and how much you eat, using advice from a dietician with an interest in functional conditions.

> Remember – it is not unusual for there to be some disruption to all your body stress systems.

This is pretty obvious so far. But some symptoms are more difficult to explain, and sometimes the disruption to the body stress systems occurred too long ago to be sure of the cause. The elements contributing to Vero's blackouts (outlined in chapter 2) only came to light after months of therapy with a trauma-informed psychologist. Vero had operated for so long by shutting down her awareness of stressors that she failed to notice the pressures increasing so much they led to blackouts. This is an extreme case of how we all can operate using denial.

Make a list of all your symptoms and try to allocate them to the body stress system involved.[23] A list of the systems and the possible symptoms are outlined in chapter 4, with a summary provided in appendix B. You may find, like Maree in chapter 8, that all systems are affected.

What factors are activating your body stress systems?

This step is vital. If you can identify the causes of your systems being activated, you can work to reduce them. So, this is a good time to write down all the stressors that have affected you recently and maybe also any stressors from your past that you feel may still be triggering a heightened response in you. Remember to check the possible factors listed in appendix B.

Identifying the causes of your symptom

With a full waiting room, your doctor may not get the time to ask you the sort of questions that would help to clarify why your symptom arose. However, if you are fortunate, your doctor would be curious about certain aspects from your functional medical history that might shed light on your situation. The following figure

---

[23] www.blueknot.org.au

outlines what these aspects might be, and how these differ from a more traditional medical history.

Traditional versus functional medical history taking

TRADITIONAL MEDICAL HISTORY	FUNCTIONAL MEDICAL HISTORY
Symptom: – when – where – what aggravates/ameliorates – past history	Symptom: – previous illness – previous life challenges – nutritional status – coexistent infections – family situation – belief systems about symptom – work, culture, environment stresses

Beyond the broader setting in which your symptoms arose, your doctor would also want to know about the following:

- What was going on in your life around the time your symptoms first arose?
- How did you feel about what was happening? How did you respond?
- What about the situation troubled you most? What did it bring up in you?
- How did you handle that? Did you seek further information and advice? From friends, family or Google?[24]

---

24 These questions have been adapted from the model outlined by Joseph Lieberman and Marian Stuart in *The Fifteen Minute Hour: Efficient and Effective Patient Centered Consultation Skills*, 6th Edition, 2019.

These questions are a preliminary probe into what is really going on for you. Answering requires time to reflect and be honest with yourself, so it's a good idea to think about them before you see your doctor, and bring up your reflections and answers even if your doctor doesn't ask. Dorothy (from chapter 6) did not initially associate her shock and dismay about her husband's infidelity with her own physical deterioration. It is not unusual for a person who cannot accept the life event to instead fixate on a symptom as a means of distracting themselves from some painful realisation. Feelings of shame, guilt, regret and loss can be hard to bear, so seeing your doctor about a health condition can be a poor substitute for the care that is lacking in your life.

Is it menopause or is it life or is it both?

Many women develop 'menopause symptoms' around the time of hormone changes. Some of these are truly helped by hormone replacement. But also at this time, women are often facing a lot of strains – possibly including elderly and needy parents, children leaving home, a shift in their identity, work and financial pressures, and the realisation that their relationship with their partner has fallen away a bit. These can all conspire to really deflate an otherwise well person. Fatigue, sleeplessness, change in mood are all common, and they don't always magically resolve with hormone therapy.

In this situation, it may help to ask what your body is trying to tell you.

When you take some time to ask yourself this question, and really consider the answers, you may find that you fully face all the events and expectations you are dealing with. Make sure you get support in dealing with this, whether that is from your doctor, counsellor or trusted friend.

And there would never be a better time for taking stock of your lifestyle. Again, a lot of people will feel better if they give proper attention to their nutrition, cut back on alcohol, get enough sleep and address the psychosocial problems that they are stressed by.

Many people have not noticed how far they have strayed from a healthy way of living, deceiving themselves that they can get away with cutting corners on these fundamental bases to good health.

No matter what the functional condition is, if you can really focus on your whole health in this way, you may be surprised how much better you feel and how the symptom may ease, if not fully resolve. But if you have been unwell for quite a while and have lost your basic level of health and fitness, you will need to be patient. It may take weeks or even months to find your vitality and lose the inner levels of tension that could contribute to your ongoing suffering.

So, a summary of steps 1 to 3 (from this and the previous two chapters) is make a note of:

- how often you are in defensive mode
- which of the seven body stress systems have been activated
- all the causes and stressors you think may be relevant.

Critically, successful treatment requires that we all, and especially my medical colleagues, work to broaden our understanding of these illnesses and their causes, remove the stigma of individual blame, and begin to find better ways to manage the symptoms.

A PROVISIONAL, NOT A FINAL, DIAGNOSIS

Whatever your symptoms, your doctor should use a systematic approach to aid in diagnosis. While tests are usually advisable to rule out possible physical causes, your doctor is usually able to make a provisional diagnosis of a functional condition from its unique characteristics. This is always what doctors do: doctors do not make a final diagnosis straightaway. It does not matter how straightforward a diagnosis might seem; doctors should always hold the thought that the diagnosis remains provisional until the agreed treatment shows improvement in your condition. Only then can we presume to make a final diagnosis.

This applies to all conditions but is highly applicable when considering your functional symptom. To ensure you have the right diagnosis, your doctor is doing several tasks:

- examining you for signs of alternate diagnoses
- observing any further changes in your condition over time that might suggest another diagnosis
- observing your response to treatment to confirm your diagnosis.

What is sometimes a problem is that doctors fail to communicate to you this routine practice. You are often left with the doubt that a functional diagnosis is not a real one. The main reason for this poor situation is the failure of medical training in the management of functional conditions. Your doctor usually has a pretty good idea about your diagnosis but might not have the training to give you a clear diagnosis, let alone outline the treatment.

Fortunately, a paradigm shift has already started. With the growing understanding of the nature of functional disorders worldwide and excellent centres bringing the research together and working according to guidelines that have been developed by hundreds of experts, more and more doctors are able to identify – and treat – these conditions.[25]

---

25 GPs like myself rely on the skills and knowledge of our specialist colleagues. As mentioned, in the case of functional symptoms, I refer to the findings and recommendations from the Mind-Body Program at Westmead Hospital, Sydney, Australia, and also utilise the latest treatment guidelines of the German College of Psychosomatic Medicine and the German Society of Psychosomatic Medicine and Medical Psychotherapy.

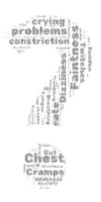

Chapter 12

Step 4: Learn how to treat your functional condition

While having any health problem is never good, the best thing about having a functional condition is that you can and should take control of your treatment back from the doctors. Now, this would not be sensible if you had a physical diagnosis – for example, a burst appendix. You would need to let the doctors do whatever it takes to save your life.

Functional conditions – however painful, disruptive or distressing they are – rarely have any effect on your longevity. But they certainly can disrupt your life and wellbeing. So it is vital that you give your condition the right amount of attention. You should be the one in control of what to do with your symptoms. You need to use your doctors and other therapists to gather as much information about what your condition is and your treatment options. Then you should be able to choose the treatment that suits you the best.

A different doctor–patient relationship

Functional conditions require quite a different doctor–patient approach, and this may feel scary at first, so be sure that you make a time to review your progress with your doctor. They should tell you the kinds of change in your symptoms that they need to hear about (red flags – refer to chapter 8). On the other hand, if you remain passive, waiting for the doctors to 'fix you', you are less likely to recover.

Before you look for treatments for your symptoms, it is valuable to examine what your approach to seeking health care is usually and what qualities are needed to become the one in control of your health.

Ask yourself these questions to determine how much you are in control of your health care:

- Do you have all your medical history gathered in one place? Typically, this would be with your usual doctor, or at least one practice.
- Have you checked with your doctor the results of all tests necessary to exclude a physical condition – that is, are you quite clear that you are dealing with a functional condition? These tests should be done once, usually. The results should be interpreted by one doctor or your team when they are all collated. This is important. (If any doubt exists about whether you could have a physical condition, it is good to run two, parallel, management strategies: the first assumes that, yes, you still could have an as yet undiagnosed physical condition and your doctor can help you exclude any possible physical condition by further testing; the second strategy assumes that your condition is functional and observes your response to appropriate treatment. If you recover with the latter, there is your answer.)
- Are you well informed about your condition? Are you aware of what may have caused it and what treatments are available for you to try?
- Do you want to join a support group of people dealing with similar symptoms?

- Have you decided about how you hope to recover from your illness?
- Do you list your priorities, in regards to all the demands on you? Sleep, work, social and family commitments, nutrition and therapy all demand your time. Try to work out what to prioritise for the best balance.
- If you choose to go to a different doctor, have you ensured that your previous history and tests have been forwarded? It is amazing what we can forget about our own health.

> **SUSI**
>
> When Susi came to see me, she was alarmed about a set of symptoms that, she told me, had just started a fortnight ago. But when I was able to show her the exact same description of symptoms in her records from three years earlier – which were found to be functional with all tests clear, with the symptoms coming and going over a short period of time – she was reassured.
>
> I cannot state too often the value of having good medical records. The Australian electronic records system, My Health Record, can be a good start – go to www.digitalhealth.gov.au/initiatives-and-programs/my-health-record for more information. You might like to make sure your records are uploaded so other doctors can access your history.

Putting yourself in the driver's seat

As you reflect on the questions just listed, you may recognise how much you have handed over the control of your health to your healthcare providers. I would encourage you to take over the responsibility for your health. Remember that having a functional condition is radically different from having a usual physical complaint, which is often best treated by your doctor, with you simply complying with the prescribed treatment or giving consent.

Once your doctor has carefully established that you do not have a physical cause for your symptoms, and has told you that you have a functional complaint, your recovery depends on you being able to understand what is causing your problem and then finding your preferred way to retrain your stress response system to switch off and allow your healthy restorative mode to take over again. After all, you have the most to gain and you know best what you want and what you have tried to date.

Sometimes, your health care is complex and needs a lot of input from numerous professionals. You need to nominate who will help you coordinate this care. GPs are well placed to assist you with this, sometimes with the help of the practice nurse. You and your GP can together write a plan that states your goals and how you expect to achieve them. Your GP can then write to the relevant health professionals and stay in communication until you are healed. That way, you and your GP can monitor your response to treatment and make the necessary adjustments.

> It is your job to make sure each member of your team is doing their part to assist your recovery.

This last statement may sound surprising, especially if you view your doctor as an authority figure who holds the power. It is true your doctor has certain powers such as writing certificates or refusing to prescribe medication they deem inappropriate, but it is useful for you to recognise your doctor's job is health care. Admittedly, sometimes in a busy practice with not enough time, this essential quality of care appears to be lacking.

Trust is not gullibility

If every time you go near a healthcare provider, a stress response is triggered in you due to a lack of trust, your path to recovery will be painfully slow. But this sounds like victim-blaming: 'You have lack of trust. If you had trust, you would be better'. Resistance to trust is understandable when you have been let down in the past, especially at a vulnerable age. You may have learnt this lack of trust as a vital survival skill at the time. The question now is whether it still serves you when you need health care and you're finding it difficult to build a trusting relationship with your team.

This barrier to treatment can be resolved and may be the first step towards recovery for you, helping you begin to build relationships without the usual stress response. Bringing a family member or friend you already trust to your consultations can help build a feeling of safety necessary for healing.

Trauma-informed therapy is very helpful in this: anyone who is recovering from trauma needs their therapist and doctor to be aware of how the simplest form of physical examination can trigger a full-blown stress response, and expectations of a good outcome are, therefore, misguided. Unfortunately, while many therapists have good skills in their area of expertise, the lack of trauma-informed training can hamper their effectiveness, to your detriment.

The Blue Knot Foundation (blueknot.org.au) has wonderful resources to assist survivors of trauma to begin the path to healing. They can help you find therapists who are trauma-informed – see appendix C for further details.

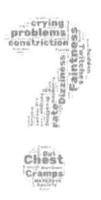

Chapter 13

Step 5: Build your team

Unlike physical conditions, which usually have a straightforward treatment regimen, your functional condition is unique and requires you to experiment with what treatment suits you best. For example, if you are having a heart attack, you go straight to the emergency department, where the nurses and doctors have the expertise to save your life. Doctors are the best trained to diagnose and treat most physical diseases, along with allied health professionals.

> It should be clear by now that once physical diseases have been ruled out, the best health worker for you is the one who can assist you to move from the defensive mode to the restorative mode, as well as assist in retraining your body to return to normal function.

Finding healthcare providers to treat your functional condition

In an ideal world, every hospital or medical clinic would have a unit similar to the Mind-Body Unit at Westmead Hospital in Sydney, dedicated to treating functional conditions, with a team of doctors ensuring no medical conditions have been missed. This would be done once but in a systematic fashion, with all the findings (or lack of them) gathered together.

Then a multidisciplinary team would meet to discuss with you the best approaches to facilitate your recovery. This may involve a dietician, psychologist, physiotherapist, exercise physiologist and doctor. Alternative health practitioners have a lot to offer in regard to re-establishing your restorative mode. The adoption of regular practices of yoga, qi gong, tai chi, simple outdoor activities in nature and breathing regulation can all serve to down-regulate your defensive mode.

Other forms of therapy, such as acupuncture, massage, aromatherapy, hydrotherapy, counselling, would also be available – anything that serves to create a place of inner calm.

However, in the real world, unfortunately, you may need to develop your own team.

A vast range of people are skilled in helping create that place of inner calm, reactivating your restorative mode. Parents with no healthcare training can often instinctively soothe their children to restore a state of calm. But a profoundly and persistently disturbed body stress system with multiple causes and symptoms may be best treated by a team of skilled professionals with an understanding of trauma, with both top–down and the bottom–up skills (see the following section), and a coordinator to ensure nothing is being overlooked.

In chapter 4, I introduced Kirralee's panic attacks and her visceral fear of heart disease. Her journey to healing took a long and, at times, unproductive route with some dead ends. Various people recommended, for example, a punishing diet or a course of vitamin injections, with dubious results. Her eventual recovery took the support of her osteopath, psychologist and GP all working together.

Many people with functional conditions find the healing work of certain alternative healthcare providers to be highly effective.

Their training is often focused on the restoration of your body stress system, getting it back to its healthy state, rather than simply targeting your specific symptoms. As mentioned repeatedly, focusing on your functional symptoms can make them worse, so a broader, fundamental approach is likely to be more beneficial.

If your doctor is dubious about the benefit of alternative healers, it may help to agree on which treatment is best to reduce your body stress system's activation. Yoga, tai chi, acupuncture and meditation have now been shown in medical studies and journals to be beneficial methods. Individual therapy can be expensive so group classes or even online therapies may be a good option.

Top-down and bottom-up approaches

Two broad care approaches are available: top-down and bottom-up. Understanding these two approaches can help you take charge of your recovery and choose the best healthcare team for you.

The top-down approach involves utilising your mental capacity to:

- understand the causes of functional conditions (reading this book is part of the top-down approach)
- learn to observe the relationship between the defensive and restorative modes and the body stress systems
- identify all the stresses, including current illnesses, nutritional deficiencies, drug and alcohol problems, mental health issues, past traumas and cultural beliefs, that could activate your defensive mode
- undertake therapy to resolve the mental and emotional stressors
- learn to recognise unhelpful mental self-talk
- accept the importance of self-compassion
- learn when to be active and when to rest.

Top-down approaches include accessing sources of information about your condition from health professionals, support groups and the internet.

The bottom–up approach is best described as finding relief from your symptoms through bodily retraining. This includes

- physiotherapy
- occupational therapy
- osteopathy
- massage
- other therapies that involve any physical means to reduce your symptoms.

The best way to initiate this approach is to adopt, as much as possible, a healthy daily routine with adequate sleep, exercise, time in nature and rest sessions. Many people with entrenched functional symptoms such as persistent fatigue need a lot of support around this because progress can seem agonisingly slow and it is easy to lose heart.

When Kirralee accepted that her heart palpitations and feelings of panic were functional, she stopped seeing cardiologists and embarked on the path to recovery by searching for the previously unacknowledged stress factors in her life. Because the cause of her nocturnal panic was not clear at the beginning, she utilised both a top–down and a bottom–up approach. She used a top–down approach with her GP and psychologist, working to address her background and personality vulnerabilities and strengths. And she used a bottom–up approach with her osteopath, who helped her get in touch with her body and notice how activated into defensive mode she was throughout the day, even though she was not aware of it previously.

Maree was also aided in her recovery by top–down and bottom–up approaches. She continues her story here, in her own words.

MAREE (continued)

I was determined that I would work my way through my symptoms, even though I didn't really understand what was happening. I had worked with lots of anxious dogs and the first thing we do is relax the nervous system. So, I did that as much as I could each day with lots of support from my husband and parents.

I started doing online qi gong[26] to help calm myself. At first, all I could do was rest and qi gong. It helped to build my confidence about being by myself in the house again and not panicking when I felt overwhelmed by symptoms.

I am very fortunate to have a neighbour who is a retired craniosacral therapist[27] who saw me weekly. I also went to a functional doctor who helped me understand what was happening in my body and make healthy changes to my diet to reduce the inflammation. The functional doctor was the first one to properly look at what had been happening over the past six years and help me realise just how much pressure I was putting on my body, combined with sleep deprivation and poor nutrition due to three pregnancies, births and breastfeeding – so it wasn't really a surprise that I was feeling so awful!

Very slowly I just kept doing a little bit more. I tried to walk my dog every day, even if it meant I could only get to the bottom of the road and then came back to rest. I also went with my mum to drop the kids off or pick them up from school when I could. I wanted to keep slowly pushing myself to do a little more each time.

That worked to an extent, but I realised after a while that I had to get rid of my rigid training mentality and stop giving myself goals to reach. It worked better to just go with what felt good on that day and be kind to myself, instead of pushing myself to get to a certain point and then beating myself up if I couldn't do it.

---

26. Qi gong, pronounced 'chi gong,' is a key part of traditional Chinese medicine. According to the US National Center for Complementary and Integrative Health, qi gong 'involves using exercises to optimize energy within the body, mind, and spirit, with the goal of improving and maintaining health and well-being' and 'has both psychological and physical components and involves the regulation of the mind, breath, and body's movement and posture'. In most forms of qi gong, breath is slow and long, movement is gentle and smooth, and attention is focused on the breath and movement or visualisation. For more information, go to www.nccih.nih.gov/health/qigong-what-you-need-to-know.
27. Craniosacral therapy is a gentle, hands-on technique used on your skull and spine to promote pain relief by decreasing tension.

Things were going quite well but I hit quite a big dip in September, so started the Gupta Program[28] which helped massively. It had been recommended by the functional doctor. The brain training has been an essential part of my recovery. The biggest lessons from the Gupta Program were recognising when my intentions/thoughts were not coming from a place that helped my recovery, and knowing how to 'float through the dips'. That also led me to the online woman's wellness circle, which helped a lot. Being able to chat with others going through something similar was very reassuring because, before that point, I did feel quite isolated.

Lots of different stepping stones have led me to new things that are still continuing now. I am feeling much stronger in my body and mind. I can keep pushing myself forwards but in a much more sustainable and healthy way, and with a lot more self-compassion and awareness of my own limits. I still have ups and downs, but I have come to realise that is life and it is our ability to float through these that helps build resilience. It has been an incredibly challenging year, but I wouldn't change it and I truly believe that it will help me live my life with more love and joy.

In fact, I have just spent a fantastic summer with my children and enjoyed it so much, especially considering how things were last summer. We also went on a weeklong trip to Ireland to visit in-laws and got stuck on the ferry for eight hours due to a technical issue! I was able to keep myself in a calm space and stay positive, which I probably would have struggled with even before I became very ill.

Maree provides us with an excellent description of what may be needed to recover from a serious functional disorder. Her motivation to be able to care for her children drove her to seek the help she needed. Her trial and error approach and capacity to learn from what didn't work for her, as well as her willingness to experiment

---

28 The Gupta Program, developed by Ashok Gupta, is a program for chronic conditions with a focus on neuroplasticity, mindfulness and holistic health. For more information, go to guptaprogram.com.

with novel approaches to her health problems, helped to guide her towards recovery.

She came to understand all the factors that had caused her previously terrifying symptoms and learnt to stop reacting with fear and instead, to listen to her body's messages without judgement and allow herself time to rest and recover. She had to learn that some of her self-talk and lack of self-compassion were perpetuating her condition. She practised meditation, which helped to reduce her habitually anxious state.

'Lose hope but keep the faith'

As well as her advice to 'float through the dips', Maree also offers the slogan, 'Lose hope, but keep the faith'. This is quite a confronting idea, and may at first seem like bad advice. And yet, when fully understood, it can help you stay the course to recovery.

If you examine your efforts to recover from your condition, you may find you experienced periods when you really felt that you had found the answer to your problem: you tried a therapy that promised so much, and it really did help. For a while, you felt great and hoped this was the cure you had been looking for. But then, your symptoms came back, and you were in despair, and you crashed. Your hopes for a cure were dashed and you found yourself feeling the situation was hopeless.

This cycle of hope followed by setbacks and subsequent emotional frustration and despondency can seriously hamper your recovery. The despair and emotional letdown can further activate your defensive mode and lead to serious setbacks.

This cycle is incredibly frustrating because you are trying so hard to get better, only to face repeated setbacks. It can feel like the situation is hopeless.

But there is a way forward. You need to adopt a subtle yet profound shift in your approach to your treatment that will lead to recovery.

> What the research shows is that one of the characteristics associated with a greater likelihood of recovery from functional conditions is the belief that recovery is possible.

This belief needs to be accompanied by holding faith in your ability to commit to the path to recovery. But this requires a new attitude that will, eventually, bring lasting results.

Fortunately, Maree was open to accepting this. Through her doctor, Maree learnt how her rigid mental attitude of pushing to her goals and hoping, by sheer willpower, that she would recover, was part of her problem. She was continually activating her defensive mode, with the consequent relapses.

She needed to abandon this pressured, goal-oriented, striving-then-collapse that had contributed to her illness cycle. And she needed to have faith that taking a new path of steadily pacing herself to stay within her limits and 'floating through the dips' would work.

This mantra, 'lose hope but keep the faith', allowed her to start each day putting in place a plan of what she could expect to achieve that day while remaining within her pacing limits, without unrealistic hopes but instead with faith in the advice of her experienced therapists. She began to see the benefit of pacing – not pushing and then collapsing, but gradually gaining more endurance. In doing so, Maree continued to 'float through the dips', which is a lovely way to express the need not to overreact with fear and self-recrimination when energies seem to flag.

As you can see, Maree became masterful at regaining her maintenance and restorative mode. Her body was finally able to heal itself and restore her energies. Her brain system was trained to recognise stressors and respond in a calm way. She trained her skeletomotor system to increase its resilience and capacity through pacing and recognising when to rest. She used mindfulness to keep her autonomic nervous system from firing up.

'I'm not nuts – why do I need a psychologist?'

When their doctor recommends they see a psychologist, the first reaction of many people with functional symptoms is to perhaps get a little defensive and wonder why this might be needed. However, psychologists have many skills beyond dealing with mental illness. As Maree showed us, you need many personal qualities to overcome a functional condition. And most of us would need some help and guidance to cultivate these qualities or learn how to apply them to beat the condition. This is especially true if, during your upbringing, you did not meet the role models or receive the parenting that would have helped you in this situation.

In chapter 2, I provide some examples that highlight the role of adverse childhood experiences and the increased likelihood of developing functional conditions in adulthood. Growing up with parents or other adults in the house who verbally, physically or sexually assaulted you, had issues with alcohol, drugs or mental health, or couldn't take care of your basic needs can all cause deep trauma. This trauma can emerge, even years later, in seemingly unrelated functional conditions.[29]

It is particularly cruel that the survivor not only endured a difficult childhood, but also continues to suffer in adulthood with physical symptoms of all kinds. Then, to make matters even more punishing, the survivor may not have been given the requisite qualities to overcome the symptoms. Coming to terms with a difficult childhood is challenging and so I advise you have good support if you need to address this.

The same is true for survivors of sexual assault. The list of long-term health problems associated with a history of sexual trauma in women is extraordinary, and includes chronic pelvic pain, premenstrual disturbance, other gynaecologic symptoms, fibromyalgia,

---

[29] For more help with this, and a questionnaire that helps you consider the impact of any adverse childhood experience, see novopsych.com.au/assessments/diagnosis/adverse-childhood-experiences-questionnaire-ace-q/.

headache, other pain syndromes, and gastrointestinal disorders.[30] The result of such trauma can damage your sense of yourself, your means of coping and your feelings about safety. Living with perpetual fight, flight or freeze response takes a lot of unlearning.

One of the features about trauma that causes ongoing difficulties is the lack of acknowledgement by those around you of your suffering. It can be a very lonely place. The retelling of your experience is an opportunity to finally be validated. This can go a long way to start your healing. Many survivors carry the legacy of low self-worth, which can create a sense that you don't even deserve to be well.

The other issue that psychologists can help you address is that some of the survival tactics, which were necessary to get through your trauma, might now be a problem in themselves. Think of Vero's collapses (outlined in chapter 2). It was only through her patient work with a psychologist that she came to realise that her survival tactic of dissociation, so successfully employed during her assaults, was no longer helping her.

It's all very well for your doctor to tell you that your symptoms are unlikely to be from a physical cause, but how do you make sense of what is a very physical experience?

Unfortunately, your doctor rarely has the time to explain what this book is seeking to outline. And even if you read this whole book, further support is usually needed.

> Your psychologist can be helpful in giving you the opportunity to really understand how this has happened to you and what you can do to recover.

---

[30] See, for example, Golding, JM (1999), 'Sexual-assault history and long-term physical health problems: Evidence from clinical and population epidemiology', *Current Directions in Psychological Science*, 8(6), 191–194.

Psychologists can help with the following:

- They can ensure you know that you are among many who have such symptoms. You are not alone.
- They can help identify any vicious cycles you may have developed. For example, they can help you see you're in a 'the more pain, the less physical activity; the less physical activity, the more pain' cycle, and help to explain how this affects your body.
- They can ensure you are clear about the bodily responses – such as trembling, tingling, or a pounding heart – that are expressions of distress (once your doctor has excluded physical causes, of course).
- They can help you learn to tolerate those internal sensations and recognise that they are both safe and tolerable.
- They can cultivate a belief in your ability to overcome urges, such as avoidance or denial. This can be immensely helpful.
- They can also help you cultivate the skill to interrupt or modify your responses – whether it is your behaviour or how you move. This helps you gain mastery over your symptoms.

Ultimately, psychologists can help you to gain what they like to call 'self-efficacy'. This allows you to overcome the reflex of triggering your defensive response whenever a symptom arises.

A psychologist can help you formulate a clear model that recognises where you are in your thinking about your symptoms, and helps you connect with possible strategies for change. For example, you might be avoiding certain activities out of fear of getting worse. Your psychologist can help you establish a safe way to move forward, addressing any concerns on the way.

One of their first tasks is to ensure you have the motivation to get better. Sometimes, it is simply a matter of making sure you believe that things can improve with a bit of effort and perseverance. But finding how to motivate you can be more complex than might appear. For example, you and your psychologist need to consider all the reasons that a subconscious process might throw up a physical symptom. I am not a psychologist, but I will say that occasionally people can develop a symptom to avoid dealing with something that, on some level, they feel is too difficult to handle. The simple example of this is the child with a tummy ache, which arises when they are afraid to go to school. Simply fixing the ache does not resolve the underlying problem.

Illness behaviour

When you first get a symptom, what do you think and what do you do? Our 'illness behaviour' is unique and has such an effect on what happens to us next that it is worth looking at this more deeply. For example, only 10 per cent of people who develop chest pain immediately seek medical attention. Most people 'try to relax', while about a third will hope and pray that it goes away. Delay in seeking help can affect your chance of survival.

When it comes to having a functional condition, your illness behaviour may make a difference between whether you recover quickly and whether your condition takes over your life. In appendix D, I include a long list of questions that can help to shape your understanding of your response to illness. These questions are not suggesting that there is a right or wrong answer, but rather can help you shape your understanding of how your symptoms are affecting you and what could be different.

These sorts of questions might come up in a consultation with a psychologist. Many of us take for granted the ideas about health and illness that we grew up with. Here is an opportunity to look at these assumptions and decide which work for you and which warrant being challenged.

Clearing the air

Sometimes doctors dump a whole lot of information on you and expect you to grasp it all. A few misconceptions after such conversations are common, particularly if the conversation was jarring.

Such a misconception might be, 'That doctor thinks this is all in my head'. A psychologist can help get across the complex ideas around your condition and help avoid simplistic and wrong notions. For example, a certain event may have been a trigger for the start of your symptoms, but not the primary cause. If you only think about the trigger, and not acknowledge all the issues that might have led to you being unwell, you may not progress.

A simple example of this is the person who bends to pick up a piece of paper on the ground and gets sudden severe back pain. The bending over was the trigger but there were almost certainly additional problems that need to be recognised. Prolonged bad posture, muscle weakness, weight gain and mental stress can all lead to a strain on the back muscles that suddenly spasm with the bending. The bending is simply the straw that broke the camel's back. A psychologist can help you work through the whole picture of your condition, as well as help you recognise the 'yellow flags' (refer to chapter 8), such as problems with your employer or the role of compensation in prolonging symptoms – the latter is a sensitive subject to raise, especially when you are suffering ongoing pain. It should only be discussed if you have the confidence the psychologist is really trying to help and not blame you.

Having a functional problem on top of a known disease is particularly difficult for you to navigate and it is helpful to be able to clarify what the different conditions are called, what symptoms they cause and what you need to do to find your path to recovery. Of course, your doctor should have explained this to you already, but these ideas are very difficult to convey in a short time and repeated consultations with both your doctor and psychologist may be needed to get this right.

For example, if you have proven epilepsy and then develop some extra symptoms that are found to be caused by psychogenic nonepileptic disorder, you will benefit from a clear set of guidelines about what should be done if you start to get certain symptoms. It also may be possible for the psychologist to help identify the extra stressors or difficulties in your life that may be contributing to the psychogenic symptoms.

Some symptoms you may have can be truly terrifying, and it does not help your recovery if you are living in fear of illness or even death every time you get your symptoms. Kirralee's terrifying night-time experiences of racing heart and feelings of dread associated with her panic attacks (outlined in chapter 4) were finally eased with the help of a good psychologist who helped her process the legacy of her childhood traumas. Kirralee needed repeated reassurance that her panic attacks, although frightening, were not going to do her any harm. She gradually learnt how to reduce and finally cease having panic attacks with the help of her psychologist.

Psychologists are well placed to help you understand what really is meant by terms such as 'psychosomatic' or 'psychogenic'. The general population and even many health professionals have a poor grasp of their real cause and the resultant responses in the body. When you really have a good understanding of why your symptoms occur, they stop controlling you and you start to control them.

During your time with your psychologist, you may recall parts of your life that were extremely difficult and perhaps your memory of these times was suppressed. Tomesia's story is an example of this.

TOMESIA

Tomesia was a very attractive woman in her late forties. She came to see me when her hospital doctor was threatening to remove her inflamed bowel. She would have had to live with a colostomy bag.

Tomesia had been dealing with being overweight for as long as she could remember. Now, her obesity was causing her a lot of problems, including knee pain. All of this caused difficulty within intimate relationships and, at times, social isolation.

Given all her stressors and the possibility of further inflaming her autoimmune bowel disease – for which she was taking maximal medication, but it was not effective – we agreed for her to have some hypnotherapy to try to reduce her defensive mode.

During one episode, Tomesia recalled a forgotten memory from when she was five years old. She could hear her mother saying she never wanted her and what a mistake it had been to have a child. Her mother then exclaimed, 'Oh, she was never meant to be born. I just wish she would disappear!'

Tomesia was shocked and then furious: *I'll show her!* thought the enraged child. And she began to eat and eat until she was enormous. And she stayed that size even when she developed a life-threatening inflammatory bowel disease. Through the regressive hypnotherapy, Tomesia was able to recall this seminal moment in her life, when she steadfastly refused to disappear and instead made herself as big as she could.

By the time we met, her mother was long dead and the need to be huge no longer had a purpose. But Tomesia had needed the therapy to recall this initial behavioural response to her mother's painful rejection. Finally, Tomesia was able to let go of her need for her oversize. She successfully lost weight for the first time in her life.

Psychologists are a vital part of your team if you want to understand your unique situation, your beliefs and fears, your unspoken hopes and dreams, your struggles and vulnerabilities – your humanness. If a psychologist is offering to work with you, it is usually worth exploring what they might be able to do.

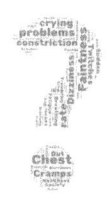

Chapter 14

Step 6: Restore your seven body stress systems

If you are living with an ongoing health problem, working to optimise the functioning of all seven body stress systems will bring you surprising benefits and is likely to resolve your symptoms over time.

Of course, this is not always easy to achieve but it is worth trying to improve your stress systems as much as possible. It should be clear from what I covered in chapters 3 and 4 that whatever has contributed to the disruption and dysregulation of your stress response systems needs to be addressed. In this chapter, I cover some ways to do so.

Autonomic nervous system: Is your environment aggravating your condition?

This is a good time to take stock of how you are living your life and try to reduce whatever is adding to your stressful mental and physical load. This may mean a reduction in your work hours or reducing the time spent with people who have a negative effect on your mental or physical health. Depending on the severity of your functional symptom, you may need to prioritise your health needs until you have settled your body stress systems and mastered the art of remaining as much as possible in the restorative mode.

Spending more time in nature is often a great place to start. Invest in clothes that keep you comfortable out of doors. Other places that have been shown to soothe the spirit are art galleries, libraries and music venues. Explore what is available to you. In Australia, you have the option of many free or affordable places to go and spend time, whether it is the local gardens or beach, or, if it is right for you, a place of worship.

Create your own sanctuary

Ideally, your home is your sanctuary, but if your home environment is noisy or upsetting and taking a toll on your wellbeing, try to find a way to change your environment to reduce the stress upon you. Create a sanctuary in your home that is clean, uncluttered and pleasing, even if this is just a corner of a shared room. Add beautiful images, flowers, candles, incense, poetry – whatever creates a sense of calm. Ideally, this space is quiet, and you should ask your house members to respect your time while in your sanctuary, because it is important for you to attend to your own needs for at least some of the day.

When you enter this space, you should feel more peaceful and able to leave the pressures of life aside, at least for a while. You might like to include a meditation space or somewhere to journal or listen deeply to music that soothes and inspires. Taking a bath or warm shower may be part of your ritual. Self-massage with a pleasant oil can be very therapeutic. Getting in touch with the *sensation* of your body, rather than *thoughts* about your body can be a powerful tool to ease the stress.

Make a habit of spending time in this space on rising and before going to bed to cultivate a state of calm and begin your journey back towards a more restful state. This means getting out of bed early enough to avoid the usual morning rush, which will trigger your defensive mode. The goal is to cultivate a deep restorative mode and then see how long you can maintain it.

Cultivating a ritual of what works for you to achieve the deepest state of calm may take a bit of trial and error, but the repetition of effective means will build an automatic triggering of calm, even before the ritual is completed. (Here the predictive processing model from chapter 5, where your brain anticipates a particular situation, will be working in your favour, so maximise this.)

Author and philosopher Alain de Botton has noted that, with our loss of religious ritual, our society has lost this habit of a dedicated time to settle our minds and focus on what is important to us. We do not need to have any particular beliefs to benefit from adopting a soothing ritual and using it 'religiously' to get the most benefit.

Understand the benefits of slow breathing

A common observation is that someone suffering from a functional condition may have a disturbed breathing pattern. As an example of this, Ethan (from chapter 4) ended up in the emergency department when he developed the complications of overbreathing. His hyperventilation was a subconscious reaction to a difficult period in his life. It took him a while to learn the art of slow breathing but he continues to benefit from this new skill.

A number of techniques enable you to master slow breathing, but a few important points should be noted:

- *Using a clock is helpful*: When you are in the defensive mode, you are automatically breathing faster so timing the length of each breath can help you realise this. Use the sweep (seconds) hand of a clock or watch rather than using a digital one.
- *Slower does not necessarily mean deeper*: You can still hyperventilate if you take very deep breaths – even if those breaths are slow – because you are exhaling excessive carbon dioxide and will continue to have your unpleasant symptoms.

One simple technique to get the benefits of slow breathing is 'box breathing':

1. Sit comfortably and inhale while counting slowly to four.
2. Hold your breath for another four counts.
3. Exhale for four.
4. Rest, holding your breath for four.

How simple is that?! Many people who suffer the symptoms of hyperventilation are breathing at a rate more than 20 breaths a minute. The box breathing rate is about six, so don't be surprised if you find it difficult at first. If you have a lung disease or another physical illness associated with breathlessness, confirm with your doctor if slow breathing is a good idea for you. But for most, the sense of not getting enough air is part of your defensive mode, which will ease with time and practice.

This conscious effort to override your defensive mode by slow breathing may be difficult initially. And if you are close to panic, it is simply not possible, so it is best to practise when you feel a little calmer, and then gradually build this bottom–up skill. (Refer to chapter 13 for more on top–down and bottom–up approaches to your recovery.)

Work on your abdominal breathing

Once you have mastered slow breathing, you may like to develop an extra technique to enhance your restorative mode – abdominal breathing. Place one hand on your chest and the other just above your navel. Your diaphragm is relaxed when breathing in the restorative mode, so focus on feeling your abdomen expand while breathing in. If you find you are holding a lot of tension in the upper abdomen and diaphragm, work on learning how to release it.

These skills were developed in the yoga traditions and are practised all over the world now. The science behind it is sound. Breathing in this way is free and you can practise several times throughout your day to gradually bring calm to your systems.

Restoring your hormonal and hypothalamic–pituitary–adrenal systems

If you have ever had difficulty falling asleep or staying asleep, it is possible that your hypothalamic–pituitary–adrenal (HPA) axis has been activated. As discussed in chapter 4, your HPA system is how your brain tells your body how to handle whatever situation you are in. It does this through chemical signals, called neurotransmitters and hormones. An important hormone that is released from your adrenal gland under all kinds of physical or psychological stresses is cortisol, which tells the body to release energy to deal with the stress.

This works well when the stress is brief, but when you remain stressed the cortisol levels will fall, leaving you feeling depleted.

Kirralee's panic attacks (refer to chapter 4) only settled when she established a daily practice of reducing the time she spent in defensive mode and allowing her HPA system to settle. She learnt about how her early experiences with violence in her home led to her adopting a perpetual state of hypervigilance – so much so that it became her default position. This meant it didn't take much to trigger her full-blown states of arousal.

Trauma-informed therapy

The lifelong impact of early childhood abuse and trauma[31] on health, behaviour and psychological patterns of response is increasingly recognised.

> It's time to stop asking, 'What is wrong with you?' and start asking, 'What happened to you?'

---

31 Examples of trauma include, but are not limited to, experiencing or observing physical, sexual and emotional abuse; childhood neglect; having a family member with a mental health or substance use disorder; experiencing or witnessing violence in the community or while serving in the military; and poverty and systemic discrimination.

Seeking forms of therapy that are trauma-informed can allow you to heal in a safe and supported environment. You will need to allow time and to keep searching for the means that works for you. Treatments proven to be effective include prolonged exposure, eye movement desensitisation and reprogramming (EMDR) and for younger people, trauma-focused cognitive behavioural therapy.

The Better Health Channel page on trauma provides information about trauma and abuse and how it changes your mind and body.[32] You will find resources, support material and counselling options. More importantly, you can find out more about the many ways to recover.

Kirralee sought help through therapy and osteopathy with trusted professionals. She no longer has panic attacks and finds her own mothering skills as she raises her beautiful little girl can work to heal her further.

When words fail to explain your trauma, various forms of art therapy can help., especially for children. Kidsxpress (www.kidsxpress.org.au), for example. uses expressive therapy to help healing.

POTS

If you nearly faint every time you stand up, it is very difficult to do much. As mentioned in chapter 4, POTS arises when your HPA system is dysregulated.

Having POTS correctly diagnosed, rather than simply saying you feel awful, is a good example of why a close working relationship with your doctor is helpful. Try to be specific regarding your symptoms – for example, explain how your heart starts to race when you stand rather than simply say you feel bad. This is easily confirmed, and then specific treatment can be given.

---

[32] https://www.betterhealth.vic.gov.au/health/conditionsandtreatments/trauma-reaction-and-recovery#reactions-to-trauma

Your treatment needs to assist you to recognise how your fear of your symptoms can make matters worse and how your focus needs to be shifted to what helps to stabilise your HPA system through returning your body to the restorative state more often.

While you pursue the best means to return to your restorative mode, you may also benefit from supportive treatments such as salt supplements, compression stockings and medication to keep your blood pressure adequate and help control your heart rate.

Your interconnected hormone system

When your hormone system is disrupted, simply replacing the required hormone is an approach that is often used. For example, a woman being in stress mode may lead to her monthly periods ceasing. Commencing the contraceptive pill may restore her monthly bleed, but this 'quick fix' does not treat the underlying issue that caused the problem.

Hopefully this book is helping you recognise how all your body stress systems closely interact and so working to improve the restorative mode in, say, your brain system will help to balance your hormone system too. Similarly, as any yoga practitioner will tell you, if you work through your skeletomotor system to reduce your defensive mode, you are more likely to see your hormones returning to their usual level.

Occasionally, hormone therapy does provide benefit and allow the other systems to recover. When Carmen (from chapter 2) was suffering her ailments, her menopausal symptoms were exacerbated and hot flushes were relentless, sending her defensive mode into overdrive. These symptoms eased when she commenced hormone replacement therapy. With fewer hot flushes disturbing her sleep, she was able to wake with enough energy to follow an exercise regime that helped to reduce her defensive mode further.

For men, a common and distressing functional symptom of hormone system disruption is the loss of sexual potency. While a number of medical conditions need to be excluded, the use of drugs such as Viagra can help couples continue to enjoy sexual relations until the man's defensive mode is down-regulated again and natural potency is restored.

So often, you will find you need to do a number of things to begin to reduce your defensive mode. Try the numerous options available. If something doesn't work, add another. Doctors and others who help people living with functional conditions take a very broad approach and it is common that several different means are needed.

Another vital role of the hormone system is the regulation of the gut. If you have a persistent activation of your defensive mode, you may struggle with digestion, which requires the timely release of hormones to stimulate your organs. Nausea, bloating and other digestive issues may arise.

You may need dietary advice to reduce the stress upon your gut, while you focus on turning your defensive mode down. Rest, especially after eating, is recommended to enhance your restorative mode. (See the section 'Microbiome–gut–brain system: It's not just what you eat, but also when and how you eat', later in this chapter, for more tips.)

Your immune–inflammatory system: Taking action to calm and restore

If you have had tests to show that your ongoing pain is not caused by a physical problem, this a terribly difficult place to be. You have real pain, but no disease or infection to treat. Taking painkillers, especially opioids, can make matters worse over time and is best avoided.

Unfortunately, this type of chronic pain can last for years unless you and your healthcare team address all the factors that are contributing to this situation. So what can you do to help free yourself from this pain?

You need to take a whole new approach to thinking about your pain. Several elements might be contributing to the perpetuation of your pain:

- You may have a dysregulated and activated immune-inflammatory system, which does several things to precipitate the experience of pain. As I cover in chapter 4, your usually very helpful macrophage cells can change from being your friendly local cleaning team to becoming rogue cells that cause inflammation and pain.
- As also outlined in chapter 4, if your brain system is also activated, your pain centres in your brain are hypersensitive to *any* message coming from your body. Your brain is on the lookout and will sometimes interpret even light touch as pain, in an effort to alert you to attack. This is helpful if you are in a dangerous place and could face injury at any moment, but usually this misinterpretation of harmless stimuli by the activated brain system is difficult to turn off.
- Your activated HPA system may have disrupted the sleep required for healing.
- All the systems being activated to keep your mind focused on your painful area will serve to intensify your awareness of pain.
- You may also have many worrying thoughts about your pain – that it may never end, for example, or could get worse or could lead to more serious health problems. All these thoughts cause increased worry and stress and lead to further activation of your body stress systems.

For you to calm and restore your immune-inflammatory system, fortunately, many of the therapeutic efforts you have already considered will help:

- Good sleep helps to achieve the restorative mode.
- Nutrition helps to reduce the inflammatory response.

- A psychologist can help you explore the way your mind responds to pain and help reduce unhelpful reactions.
- Getting help from a physiotherapist, occupational therapist or exercise physiologist with an interest in chronic pain can help to restore good functioning. Their techniques can also help to reduce your pain.

If you want to understand more about pain (and you would if you are putting up with it without understanding it), Professor Lorimer Moseley's website is a great place to start – go to www.painrevolution.org. If you think you understand pain, be prepared to be surprised. Pain clinics can be helpful too.

I discuss the role of medication in the next chapter, but note that a strong effort should be made to address any factor that may be affecting your body stress systems, because this may play a role in creating and maintaining your general wellbeing.

Circadian rhythm: Establish a regular sleep–wake cycle and let your sleep start to heal you

If you have a problem with a functional symptom, it is common to also have difficulty getting a good night's sleep. Conversely, if you work on getting a good night's rest as a priority, you are on your way to improving your health. Remember that the deep phases of sleep are the ultimate restorative mode, and much of your body's repair and rejuvenation happens then. So, particularly if you have a disrupted body stress system, your circadian rhythm needs to be prioritised.

Many people struggle with getting enough sleep. Or their sleep–wake cycle is very irregular. As I mention in chapter 4, your circadian rhythm is not only vital for your good health, but also often disrupted as part of your stress response. Many of your symptoms may be aggravated by poor sleep habits so it is worth your while working to improve your circadian rhythm.

Choose a bedtime and wake time that suits your schedule and ensures adequate sleep – and then try to stick to it. It can take some time to establish this routine. Slowly move your bedtime back by 15 minutes daily to allow your body clock to readjust. Dr Kasia Kozlowska offers some further tips in the following box. (Note that Dr Kozlowska's work is focused on children but her tips on improving your circadian rhythm apply equally to adults.)

> **SHIFTING THE CIRCADIAN CLOCK BACK TO A NORMAL, HEALTHY RHYTHM**
>
> The human sleep cycle, which follows the 24-hour circadian clock, can shift itself only about two hours a day (equivalent to two time zones). When trying to move away from a very disrupted sleep cycle – for example, a reverse sleep cycle of sleeping during the day – some children prefer to reset their clocks gradually by going to bed two hours later each day until the targeted sleep time is reached. Going to bed earlier (for example, by two hours each day) generally does not work. Alternatively, it is much faster and also potentially easier for the child to accumulate sleep debt by staying up all day, all night, and all of the following day, and to then go to bed at the targeted time.[33]

If these tips on changing your sleep routine don't work, discuss with your doctor the role of melatonin or other medication.

Shift workers deserve a special mention here, and often have difficulty with the establishment of a healthy circadian rhythm. If your functional condition is serious, it might be worth changing jobs, if possible, to ensure your vital restorative work is achieved.

Prioritise your sleep

If your health is very poor and you are dealing with very troubling functional symptoms, or you are fed up with your aches and pains,

---

[33] Kozlowska, K, Scher, S, Helgeland, H & Chrousos, G (2020), *Functional Somatic Symptoms in Children and Adolescents: A Stress-System Approach to Assessment and Treatment*, Palgrave Macmillan.

then consider the following radical approach: that you aim to structure your life to achieve one goal – a good, deep sleep. Sleep is so important for your recovery that it deserves your careful consideration. Many people use the time that should be allocated for sleep as if it is optional, and that sleep time can be taken over by work, gaming or social engagement.

Others would like to sleep but find their mind racing and their nights full of an army of thoughts marching through their mind, disrupting any effort to sleep. Sleep disorders such as obstructive sleep apnoea or restless leg syndrome can play havoc with the time you should be resting and healing. Drugs and alcohol and caffeine can also disrupt your sleep. PTSD sufferers often face nightmares when they sleep.

How do you know if you are getting enough quality sleep?

- You wake around the same time without an alarm.
- You feel refreshed and energised.
- You don't need caffeine and other stimulants to get going.
- Your mood is good.

Sounds good, right? Let's see what can be done to achieve this.

Restoring your circadian rhythm to optimise your chances of healing

Start by choosing the time you need to get up so that you are not rushing in the morning. Then count back the hours from this time to ensure you get a solid eight or so hours' sleep. Then mark the time that you need to set aside in the evening to prepare for sleep. This is the time you should set an alarm for! (As mentioned, if you are getting enough sleep, and have established a good circadian rhythm, you should wake spontaneously without an alarm.) So, this time in the evening needs to be clearly defined as the time when all the demands in your life are put aside, and you focus on what you need to ease your mind into a deep sleep. Consider things like a warm shower, a quiet read, a herbal tea, some soothing music or sleep-inducing podcasts. Make sure you allow yourself this prioritising of an important part of your day.

If you believe that you do not have the time for this reprioritising of your time, like Maree, you might like have a talk to your internal slave-driver: you may have to postpone that extra study or the second job until your health is restored. Leave the office on time. Guard the use of your precious time and make sure to discard anything that puts you in defensive mode and is not essential.

> If you are spending much longer than eight hours a day in a form of work that activates your defensive mode, then you cannot expect to achieve a deep restorative mode when it comes time to sleep.

However, you may be trying to fall asleep at the right time, but it eludes you. Have a look at the quaintly named 'sleep hygiene' guidelines from the Victorian Government's Better Health Channel (details provided in appendix C). If sleep remains a problem, you may need to use a sleep psychologist. Sometimes, despite all efforts, you may require medication such as melatonin or other medication to reduce your anxiety or pain enough to sleep.

Skeletomotor system

Your muscles are a common source of functional symptoms, when they react to a heightened defensive mode. A good example is Min's tight throat, or globus, from chapter 2. Min struggled to accept that the alarming and new sensation of her throat closing was functional, even after physical causes such as reflux or other structural issues had been explored and ruled out by careful internal examination.

In this situation, a speech therapist can help to explain that globus occurs more often in response to muscles of the larynx and throat becoming tight – especially if the person had been under a lot of pressure, possibly worrying about things, or dealing with feelings of sadness or worry that had been difficult to talk about. Having introduced these ideas as possibilities, the therapist can then explain that this can lead to the larynx being held rather high in the neck, leading to a feeling of limited space and difficulty swallowing. With some gentle manoeuvres to lower the larynx, they can relieve the tight muscles holding the larynx. This can create more of a feeling of space, swallowing becomes easier, and the symptoms can gradually disappear.

Of course, because this throat tightening is reflexive, it is likely to recur if the underlying pressures and perhaps unrecognised emotions are not dealt with. Many people opt to live with their functional symptom rather than deal with the possible causes.

With greater recognition of the reality of functional conditions by the community, it is my hope that people like Min don't have to suffer and, instead, a prompt acceptance of these commonplace phenomena leads to conversations that open the door to expressing feelings that might have been bottled up for some time.

Other symptoms caused by the skeletomotor system can be varied, but many are eased by increasing gentle physical activity.

Are you getting enough daily physical activity?

As I outline in chapter 4, physical activity helps to switch your defensive mode to restorative mode and facilitate your path to healing. But to get the benefit of the physical activity, you need to do it regularly. Note that I'm not talking about intense exercise or sport. It is not necessary to work yourself to the bone to gain the benefit of activity. You merely need to be mildly breathless while exercising – for example, walking briskly. If this is too difficult for you at this stage, start where you are and try to maintain a short spell of activity a few times a day.

Exercise physiologists are a fabulous resource to help you pace yourself, encourage progress and identify any problems that could impede you gaining more fitness. It is a good idea to attend to their advice, so your recovery is not set back by excessive efforts or injury, and so you are given realistic expectations as to when to expect a return to normal activity.

Once you know what you can do, several apps are available that can help you on your way and keep you motivated.

If you are going to do this on your own, start with a list of forms of physical activity that you think you could enjoy. It is helpful to do this with a friend, because they can help you through any resistance that will inevitably arise. Try out a few different forms of movement, which may include anything from simply taking a walk to taking classes in yoga, dancing or tennis. Swimming is great for many reasons – see the section, 'Taking the plunge', later in this chapter, for more on why.

Other forms of activity include qi gong and tai chi, both of which emphasise relaxed movements that can provide health and fitness benefits, and help your body return to restorative mode.

Let's get physical

No matter what your functional symptom is, it will often improve if you keep moving. Any physical activity that you can do and especially that you enjoy can help. The study of the benefits of exercise has changed how we think about healing. In my lifetime, heart attack patients were ordered to have strict bedrest for weeks. But now they are encouraged to get moving within a day sometimes!

This is a good time to recognise all the benefits of exercise that you are potentially missing out on. In broad terms, regular physical activity can help improve your sleep, reduce anxiety and lower blood pressure. Over the long-term, it has been shown to improve brain and heart health, increase bone strength and even reduce the risk of cancer.

More specifically, research shows regular workouts can:
- build agility
- decrease your risk of metabolic syndrome
- delay onset of dementia
- give you more confidence

- improve creativity
- improve fertility
- improve your posture
- improve your skin
- increase your energy
- increase your flexibility and range of motion
- lower your risk of injury
- make your DNA younger
- reduce back pain
- reduce chronic pain
- reduce stress
- relieve PMS symptoms
- strengthen your joints
- support your eye health.[34]

To see progress with whatever exercise you choose, the old adage 'The more you put in, the more you get out' holds. It's best to have a daily program, and preferably repeated bouts of different types of physical activity throughout the day.

Using a graded approach

Aches and pains may make you feel like physical activity is the last thing you want to do, so this is where a *graded* exercise program is recommended. Here's how to get started:

1. First, try to find an activity that you like – or at least dislike the least! Look for something that is available, affordable and scalable – by 'scalable' I mean something that you can slowly increase, either in time spent on the activity or distance. Walking is the simplest but if you are struggling to find an activity you can manage, finding an exercise physiologist is a very helpful idea.
2. Then, starting *very* modestly, do a brief session.

---

[34] For more ways exercise can improve your health, see www.piedmont.org/living-real-change/25-ways-exercise-can-change-your-life.

3. Wait until the following day to assess the effect. If you feel worse, you may have done too much, so half your training period for the next session.
4. Repeat this review after your next session.

Keep the following in mind:

- If you find you managed the session quite well, or certainly you didn't feel worse, try increasing by only five to 10 per cent. So, if you managed a walk for 10 minutes, only increase it to 11 minutes.
- The goal is to gradually increase your exercise period, remembering that even if you are active for an hour a day, you are still sedentary for just less than 96 per cent of the day!
- You may need to do two or three briefer sessions through the day while you build your tolerance.
- Try to exercise every day and then reassess after three weeks. After this amount of time, you will see the impact.

This slow, graded return to physical activity can be very rewarding. But go slowly to avoid injury.

Taking the plunge

Swimming, hydrotherapy or aquarobics are fabulous activities for those with pain and weakness. It helps increase muscle strength and cardiovascular fitness, and by taking some of the impact stress off your body, can be particularly good for people with functional conditions.

> No matter how sick or weak you are, the benefits of hydrotherapy, or water-based activity, are simply wonderful. Moving in water has remarkable benefits for the body ... and soul!

Look for hydrotherapy opportunities near you – your local swimming pool or aquatic centre is a great place to start, and many offer pool-based low-impact group classes.

Another option you may have heard of is cold-water therapy. This has its proponents, although the evidence is not yet great. Sudden exposure to very cold water can massively over-stimulate your defensive mode and should not be done without guidance and training. No data on its effects on functional conditions is available at the time of writing.

Microbiome–gut–brain system: It's not just what you eat, but also when and how you eat

So much advice is available about diet these days, it is easy to be overwhelmed and give up. The evidence for the latest trendy diet is often very poor, but that doesn't mean you should ignore some commonsense approaches that will improve your health.

Your doctor would encourage you to adopt a simple nutritional plan that includes all the major food groups, good sources of vitamins and minerals, and plenty of fibre to aid the gut function and improve your gut biome – that is, the healthy bacteria that play a role in how your whole body functions, including your brain and nervous system. Evidence is mounting that processed foods disrupt the health of the gut biome (the DNA of healthy bacteria) and this can affect mental and physical health.

No one diet suits all, and certain conditions would necessitate dietary modification, so get good advice from your doctor or qualified dietician.

The improvement in your health when you attend to your dietary needs may take several weeks to manifest so make sure you persevere. Trust the science that has shown again and again how important good nutrition is.

Which is the best diet?

The truth is we don't know which diet is the best. But some simple rules apply to whatever diet you choose:

- *Variety*: To get enough of the vast number of nutrients that benefit the human body, it is good to include a range of different foods in your diet. Nutrient-rich foods, such as nuts and seeds, peas and beans, and eggs should be part of your diet, unless you have reasons to avoid them.
- *Moderation*: Worldwide, people clearly have a problem with this, with nearly 40 per cent of the world population overweight. Humans are overeating for many reasons, and overcoming this is clearly very difficult. We need to battle some powerful forces to keep the waistline in check.
- *Balance*: When it comes to food, it is best to avoid simplistic thinking – such as, because a food item is considered good for you, you can eat as much of it as you want. Focus instead on healthy portions of each group.

If you want a good starting place, the Mediterranean diet[35] ticks all the boxes for a healthy diet. Again, individual needs still should be taken into account so chatting with your GP or a dietician is worthwhile.

Remember – you could be eating the most well-balanced diet designed for your needs and still suffer from gut disturbance. This is where the brain may be influencing the gut, not just vice versa (see the following section).

Also have a look at when and how you eat. An important aspect of the Mediterranean diet is enjoying your food with others. Doing so can not only improve social connection and happiness, but also

---

35 A Mediterranean diet includes lots of vegetables, fruits and legumes, olive oil as the principal source of fat, fish at least twice a week, moderate amounts of poultry, diary and eggs, and small amounts of red meat and sweets. For more information, and a handy diet pyramid, see memory.ucsf.edu/sites/memory.ucsf.edu/files/MediterraneanDietHandout.pdf.

encourage more mindful eating and healthier choices. Do you slow down and really taste and smell the good things you are eating? Pausing to savour your food aids the stimulation of your restorative mode and allows you to start to digest your food in a healthier fashion. In contrast, eating while on the run means that your defensive mode is trying to prepare your body for some threat and this is certainly not conducive to aiding your digestion: you can expect nausea and digestive disorders.

Hint: If your mouth is often dry, you may have activated your microbiome–gut–brain stress system and turned off the normal digestive responses.

Your relationship to food is an important part of your recovery. Doctors know that raising the issue of unhealthy nutritional problems of over- or under-eating can add to feelings of shame and guilt which, of course, can trigger the defensive mode. This delicate situation is best dealt with on your terms. Free resources such as the fellowships of Overeaters Anonymous or the Butterfly Foundation (see appendix C) can provide the support you need to work towards a healthier relationship with food.

Your brain system: Looking after your mental health

If you are living with an ongoing health problem such as a functional condition, it is totally understandable that you may suffer from some anxiety or depression. It is also possible that your mental health itself is contributing to your stress response and consequent symptom load.

As I outlined in chapter 4, the body stress systems get activated when mental problems such as anxiety, stress or panic arise. All these systems interact with the brain. The capacity for the body to rejuvenate and repair itself, for example, requires a healthy circadian rhythm, and this is often disrupted with mental illness. The capacity for you to get good nutrition and exercise can also be difficult.

How to optimise your brain system to remain in restorative mode

Your body returning to, and remaining in, restorative mode requires calm. Allow time to enjoy quiet periods with yourself, right from when you wake up. Whether it is a walk, sitting in meditation or listening to music or birdsong, try to start the day in the right space.

As your day passes, check in with yourself and note all the things that might contribute to a poor sleep and stressed mental state – for example, unresolved conflicts, work pressures, use of caffeine, drugs and alcohol, the amount of physical activity you get, and eating late in the day. Writing them all down can be quite a revelation.

The Yerkes-Dodson curve is a useful tool for you to track your status. The following figure shows a version of this curve, adapted to bring in your body's restorative and defensive modes. The curve shown on the figure is the usual response to demands on us: the greater the 'output' or performance requirements, the greater the stress, until we start to fail under the strain.

Yerkes-Dodson curve and the restorative and defensive mode

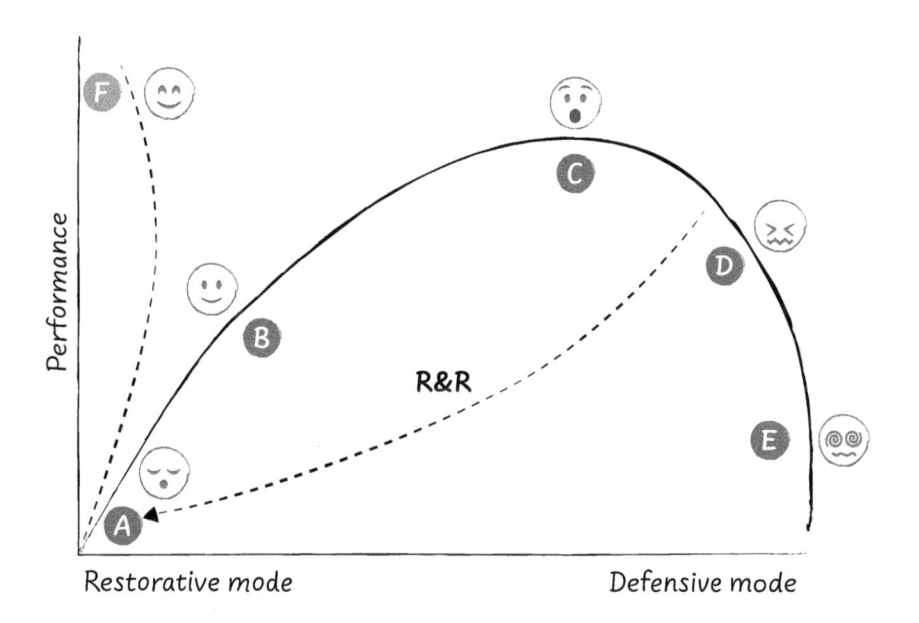

Here's what the other points shown on the Yerkes-Dodson curve relate to:

- A marks your resting state – no performance but restful.

- B is the usual place you can operate from for prolonged periods with good output and minimal stress. On the Yerkes-Dodson curve, this is your comfort zone.

- C is peak performance. Yes, the stress levels are high – you are in 'stress mode' – but you are sprinting to achieve your goals. This is the growth and learning zone.

- D is where you can start to slide. While some of us try to stay at peak performance all the time, this state is unsustainable over the long term. You begin to feel fatigue, your temper starts to fray, you make mistakes and illnesses can occur more frequently. This is the distress zone.

- E is burnout and breakdown, and this is where you can end up if you try to stay on despite the warning signs from point D. At this point, you are quite unwell and struggling to carry on. The Japanese have a word for this end stage: 'karoshi', or death from overwork. This is when a worker dies tragically young after working under extreme conditions of long hours without a break or under intense pressure. Karoshi is the ultimate functional condition (mercifully rare).[36]

You may be interested in the second curve shown on the figure. This is where a very high level of performance is achieved while remaining in the restorative mode. This curve, showing you can work and live while remaining in the restorative mode, is achieved

---

36 The other neologism related to this area is also Japanese. 'Karajisatsu' is suicide from overwork or stressful working conditions. While credit can be given to the Japanese for at least naming, and so acknowledging this phenomenon, it remains an appalling situation.

through developing mindfulness throughout your day, starting with sessions of mindfulness training to help you get in touch with your day-to-day operating mode. Gradually you will notice what state you are in and what triggers your defensive mode.

You will also need to practise some means of reducing your stress response through the day, whether you use a breathing technique or a mantra, or simply taking some time out to sit in nature. The goal is to spend most of your day in your restorative mode, with occasional 'stress mode' episodes that are self-limiting – for example, with physical activity followed by rest. (Remember, your stress mode is perfectly normal and indeed essential, but you need to learn how to keep it in check.)

Initially, you may find that you will only be able to maintain your restorative mode when you are doing very little, but gradually you should be able to master the skill of remaining calm and focused, with minimal stressors, even as you work. This is represented as point F on the figure, and has been called the 'high functioning' or 'executive' state, or 'flow'. The more time you can attain this state of calm, the more likely that your functional symptoms will begin to abate.

However, this state of achieving high performance while remaining calm is very advanced, and most of us do well simply remaining between points A, B and C. It is important that you build enough resilience and awareness to move comfortably with the occasional bit of stress.

Avoidance is not the goal

Keep a keen eye on the goal of returning to an engaged, interactive, productive life, with only brief moments of stress that you can manage skilfully. It is tragic when people 'solve' their problem by retreating ever further from life. This is where therapy can be useful.

Maree's story (outlined in chapters 8 and 13) is proof that recovery from severe and disabling symptoms is possible, with the support of professionals skilled in training you to master your stress response, using whatever means possible. Over the years, many techniques have been developed. It is important that you evaluate the results of your new practices over the weeks and months required to retrain your body stress systems. Keep in mind Maree's exhortation to 'lose hope but keep the faith' as you persevere through the good and bad days towards your goal.

Don't be dismayed to find yourself frequently at point D or even point E on the Yerkes-Dodson curve, despite your efforts.

> Your symptoms may flare in the most exasperating and inexplicable way. Don't lose heart. This is normal on the path to recovery – after all, you may have spent a long time 'hardwiring' your stress response.

Remember also Maree's advice to 'float through the dips' (from chapter 13). This is represented on the curve as 'R+R', or rest and recreation. Remember that it probably took years to reach the threshold where your functional symptoms emerged, so they won't disappear overnight.

So, take the pressure off yourself, have a break, find something enjoyable or creative to engage you and stop you focusing on your symptoms. And, provided you keep in check your worry and fears – anything that aggravates your defensive mode – you will find that you can recommence your journey to recovery once more.

Maree needed to find new sources of support as she met different barriers. She learnt more about herself and was able to develop new life skills and have less anxiety than she had ever had.

Understanding neuroplasticity and making it work for you

You may know how the neurones in your brain learn to do things automatically, by frequent repetition. Think of the difference between the first time you tried to write your name and now!

Now try to write with your other hand: most of us are not 'hard-wired' to do this, so it is slow and clumsy. But repetition would gradually change your brain to adopt a more automatic style.

The same goes for your new way of being: you may understand the task, but find it frustratingly slow to rewire your brain. It may help to imagine your automatic skills as a wide highway you can drive down at speed and with ease, whereas going a new way is similar to hacking a new path in the jungle. Initially, progress is slow and only repeated journeys make it easier.

Are you a 'heartsink' patient?

The pernicious effect of mental illness cannot be ignored, even if you have a character that can withstand the burden of mental illness without complaint. Many people with mental illness have an extraordinary capacity to endure the suffering without seeking help. Some of them are under the illusion that mental illness is a sign of weakness and should never be admitted. They can, however, believe that physical symptoms can and should be treated. Doctors have a word for these patients: 'heartsink' patients. These patients (and so their doctors) are caught in a bind: their focus is fixed on their endless physical complaints and yet they fail to recognise all the sources of malaise that may have produced them.

If your focus has been on how to diagnose or treat your physical symptoms, this may be a frustrating experience and potentially could aggravate a mental health problem. You may even have a sense you are a 'heartsink' patient as your doctor's attitude towards you is ... different. Doctors struggle to deal with this clinical problem: they cannot cure the symptoms, because the underlying problem is not recognised, either by the doctor or the patient. Your doctor may seem frustrated, dismissive or simply unsure what else to do for you. Doctors often will try to just listen to what is going on for you but the real issue – that of the disruption to your stress response systems – is not discussed. Whatever treatment is offered is not effective, but if your doctor tries to raise issues outside your presenting symptom, you may not have been ready to explore these issues, such is your focus on the immediate concern of your physical symptom.

The frustration will be mutual and often a heartsink patient will go from one doctor to another in a futile search for the solution they are willing to accept. Given functional symptoms arise out of a disrupted body stress system, they will change in character and intensity over time, so some response may seem to arise from a suggested treatment option, only to fail shortly after.

It is well known that many people with mental health issues will carry a significant burden of physical complaints too. These various symptoms will often lift when all your stressors – internal and external – are dealt with. Some people will primarily *somatise* their problem – that is, they will express it through bodily symptoms. We have English phrases that reflect this: 'heartache' or 'nauseating' or 'pressured'. Stressors, by definition, affect our bodies. (If they don't have a physical impact, they are not stressors.) Is it possible the link is being ignored by you?

Provided you have been given the reassurance that your symptoms are not the result of a physical illness – that is, they are likely to be functional – it would be in your interest to shift your focus from them and prioritise addressing all the possible sources of stressors.

You should keep in touch with your doctor and report any changes that concern you, but you may be pleasantly surprised when, through addressing *all* the sources of your stressors, your good health is restored.

How do you identify the sources of stressors? One of the best ways is to just start writing a list of all the things in your day that cause any aggravation, fatigue, irritation, frustration or unpleasant physical symptoms, no matter how small. It may be that you don't get enough sleep, or your relationship with your boss makes you feel sick. It might be your relentless perfectionism or the fact you always feel judged. Maybe your self-criticism never lets up.

Many people have benefited from seeing a psychologist or a psychiatrist, who can help to source the problems that are activating your body stress system.

Online mental health apps, most of which are free or reasonably affordable, can be very helpful too. Black Dog Institute can get you started with some good research-backed options – go to www.blackdoginstitute.org.au/resources-support/digital-tools-apps to check them out.

Other causes of functional conditions

Factors such as poor job satisfaction or an overprotective family have been shown to increase your likelihood of ongoing symptoms. Could these kinds of common life events be triggering your defensive mode? It doesn't take much to see how a negative work environment affects your day-to-day functioning. And a family culture of fear of harm or one that makes excessive efforts to avoid risk can create an atmosphere of hypervigilance, which (as discussed) can trigger the sympathetic system into overdrive.

Your psychologist can help you to recognise this pattern and learn strategies to reduce your state of arousal. Of course, health often improves when you move from a toxic environment, whether this is work or home.

Summary of the journey ahead

Here's a summary of how you can move from the defensive mode to the restorative mode:

- Cultivate a calm atmosphere to avoid triggering your autonomic nervous system reflexes.
- Restore your hormone levels optimal for the restorative mode to re-establish. Note any disruption to hormonal function as a sign of possible resurgence of defensive mode.
- Understand the complexities relating to the immune-inflammatory system, recognising that pain and inflammation

are among some of the symptoms, and apply a systematic approach using one of the well-recognised methods of treatment for chronic pain.
- Optimise your circadian rhythm and quality of sleep.
- Find the right form of physical activity that builds your resistance but optimises your restorative mode.
- Choose the diet that nourishes your biome and eat with minimal stress activation.
- Address all the factors that led up to you developing a functional symptom. (This may include early childhood trauma.)
- Recognise where you are on the Yerkes-Dodson curve and take measures to be productive while still mostly staying in the restorative mode.

The preceding points provide a very broad list of principles that apply to most functional conditions. Writing a plan for your recovery that includes an action on each of these eight aspects, focusing on the area most relevant to you, can be very helpful. For example, your nutrition might be fine but your sleep terrible, so you need to prioritise sleep (using the strategies mentioned in this chapter and resources listed in appendix C).

In the next chapter, I take a quick look at the three categories of functional disorders and what therapies may be considered. The purpose is to give you a taste of how to approach your problem. I use a few examples of each category to illustrate the approach.

Chapter 15

A few examples from each category to illustrate treatment options

This book provides an overview of functional conditions, and a potential approach to your problem. I encourage you to seek a deeper explanation of your condition and its treatment, with a word of warning: if you search 'functional medicine' online, websites that promote various supplements and other expensive and unproven therapies will likely come up in your search. Utilising *any* therapy that brings you benefit is worthwhile, but remember Maree's advice to 'lose hope but keep the faith' – that is, don't look for a quick fix but commit to a regular daily program that will gradually bring improvement in your wellbeing, despite the occasional setback.

In chapter 2, I outline the three categories used to describe the degree of impact of function symptoms. These categories are:

- *persistent functional **symptoms*** that are ongoing and may impair how you function in some way
- *functional somatic **syndromes*** that have a defined group of symptoms, recognised and treated by doctors

- *somatic stress **disorders***, which are associated with multiple symptoms and are the most disabling.

Given the vast array of functional conditions, in this chapter I focus on pointing you in the right direction for possible treatment options for your symptoms. Appendix C also has a number of resources that you may find useful.

Treatment for persistent functional symptoms

This group of conditions all share a functional cause but have other factors that lead to you getting one condition and not another.

Hyperhidrosis

I mention excessive sweating, or hyperhidrosis, in chapter 2. Those who suffer this condition know that it is often aggravated by the stress of some social interactions. While addressing any underlying social anxiety may be helpful, trialling a potent antiperspirant to the sweaty area every night for a few weeks can be effective. If this isn't enough, then Botox can be tried. If this also fails, then the sympathetic nerve can be cut – drastic but effective.

Globus

Globus was mentioned in chapter 2 as an example of a persistent symptom. The unpleasant sensation of your throat tightening can be aggravated by your activated body stress systems, especially your autonomic and skeletomotor systems. So, anything that aids the return to your restorative mode will help. But sometimes, due to activation of your microbiome–gut–brain system, you have acid reflux rising from your stomach and irritating your throat – a galling situation! So anti-reflux measures can also aid your recovery.

*

Many persistent functional symptoms can be ameliorated by medication. It is best not to have a rigid ideological attitude for or against medication, but keep in mind your real purpose is to regain your health. The *ultimate* goal would be to try to cease medication but sometimes it is very useful in the early stages. (See the section 'The role of medication', later in this chapter, for more in this area.)

As also discussed in chapter 2, Min (eventually) turned to a speech pathologist to help her with her globus. If you are reading this far, you may have already accepted your diagnosis may be functional. From here, the treatment choices lie with you. Even if it takes time and progress seems slow (or even non-existent), be reassured that your body is fine and your path to recovery will be unique to you.

So, go ahead and enjoy learning what works for you. You will know yourself better after this.

Treatment of the functional somatic syndromes

Many functional conditions have internationally recognised treatment guidelines. Your doctor is familiar with these, and I won't go into them here, except to say if you have one functional condition, you may have more. This is quite common.

But many of the guidelines are highly medically focused and fail to state the importance of modifying the defensive mode. The best approach is often to use both the medical treatment and the broader approaches described in this book.

> Whatever your condition, never lose hope that, with the right approach, you can improve your health and wellbeing.

Headaches

Headaches are a common feature of functional illnesses. Many factors contribute to you getting headaches, and these include sleep disturbance, dehydration, stressors of any form, certain foods, especially alcohol, and a history of migraine (which can lead to ongoing headaches).

Identifying the triggers that are the connection between your headache and you being in defensive mode can take considerable effort – whether the trigger is the wrong food chemical, activating the microbiome–gut–brain system, or a fight with your mother-in-law, activating the brain system, or grinding your teeth, activating your skeletomotor system. (Grinding your teeth, or bruxism, is a surprisingly common cause of headache.)

While medication can certainly help, seeking to understand your triggers requires a headache diary, where you document all the possible causes. For women, this includes tracking their menstrual cycle because the hormone system is frequently involved.

As you can see, all body stress systems can play a role in headache. See appendix C for online resources that really help.

Irritable bowel syndrome

Similarly, irritable bowel syndrome (IBS) can be aggravated by multiple body stress systems. The most obvious one is the microbiome–gut–brain axis, where certain foods can trigger your symptoms of bloating, discomfort and disturbance to your bowel function. But the activation of the brain system and the autonomic nervous system through lifestyle triggers such as eating on the run or when in a psychologically activated state is often overlooked as a contributing factor.

Medication can modify your symptoms, but a focus on your diet, particularly addressing the link to the 'FODMAP' foods (see appendix C for more resources in this area), as well as developing a way of living compatible with remaining in restorative mode, can be very helpful.

Treatment of the functional persistent disorders

Functional persistent disorders are the most complex. As you saw from Maree's story (from chapters 8 and 13), it may take multiple different forms of therapy to recover from these sorts of disorders. This is definitely an area where medicine could do a lot better. It is rare for you to get a timely diagnosis, let alone have a team available to assist your recovery. Some good online sources of information about functional neurological disorders are available, such as such as FND Hope (fndhope.org) and FNDAus.org.au.

You are likely to need to develop your own team. This book can serve as a guide to encourage a different approach to your health problem. Work with your doctor and get support as you navigate the various means by which you seek to recover and stabilise your restorative mode. This will take a daily, almost hourly, commitment and often multiple methods.

As Maree found, you will likely make progress and then suffer some setback, and so need to re-evaluate your approach. Again, any setback should be acknowledged, and your response discussed with your doctor.

The role of medication

Most of this book has focused on describing to you that your perfectly normal body has a glitch in its functioning that causes your symptoms. Sometimes the severity of the symptoms can cause a fear in you that something must be wrong that warrants medication, antibiotics or even surgery. If your condition is purely functional, the focus needs to be on how best to restore normal functioning. So, does medication have a role?

Certainly, all your therapeutic options are worth considering, and medication is one of them. For example, if your condition includes pain, medication that reduces the strength of the messages being transmitted to your brain can be helpful. Amitriptyline is one example of potentially useful medication.[37] This medication can help to confirm to you that the diagnosis is correct when your symptoms ease. This is deeply reassuring and allows you to commit to the journey of reprogramming your body stress systems without the fear that something has been missed. Existential fear is a powerful stimulant of the defensive mode, so being able to let go of fear of disease and move your focus towards what it takes to return to restorative mode can be extremely beneficial.

When your circadian rhythm is badly disrupted and you are struggling to restore it, melatonin can help. Generally, sleeping pills such as the benzodiazepines are best avoided because of the risk of addiction and other problems. Pain medication has a role to play, but it is best to avoid opiates because they usually cause more trouble than they solve.

As mental health problems such as anxiety and depression can contribute to you developing functional symptoms, treatment for these is likely to help reduce functional symptoms. This may include medication, but you should work closely with your doctor to ensure you gain the most benefit.

Because functional illnesses are more common in those with existing physical conditions, knowing when to treat each requires considerable skills. For example, the epileptic patient who develops functional seizures needs to know how much anti-epileptic medication is required for their epilepsy, while engaging in other forms of treatment for their functional seizures.

A disturbance in your gut microbiome may require treatment with medication but this area is generally poorly understood and excessive reliance on medication is not likely to help.

Serious functional conditions such as takotsubo cardiomyopathy (refer to chapter 4) need urgent treatment to take the strain of

---

37 These drugs were first created to treat anxiety and depression, but when taken at a low dose, amitriptylines can also be useful for treating pain, especially nerve pain.

massive adrenaline release off the heart. Then the treatment focus should be on what 'broke' your heart.

Panic attacks are often treated with medication to settle the severe symptoms, but long-term use of medication can be counterproductive.

> In most cases, medication may mitigate your symptoms, but is not the cure.

What is clear is that a mutually respectful relationship with your doctor is necessary to try to resolve your symptoms. No one quick fix is usually possible, and you may need to try several methods to heal. Work with your team and communicate your results, moving forward each time. A failure of treatment is still helpful in that it tells you what direction to turn to next.

Conclusion

Functional symptoms need to be recognised for what they are: the bodily expressions of our activated stress response systems. Once your doctor has ensured that nothing is wrong with your physical body, you can be confident to move towards a new understanding of how your symptoms arose.

Learning to recognise whether you are in restorative and maintenance mode or defensive mode is a great start. Identifying all the stressors that can activate your defensive mode then allows you to begin the work to allay them. At the same time, you now know that a sustained effort to establish a daily lifestyle that is conducive to restorative mode is necessary for healing to take place.

Getting the right help through your doctors, allied health professionals and other practitioners as well as support groups and online resources will go a long way to restoring your natural state of health. Given how poorly understood these conditions are, you may need to provide resources such as this book to those trying to support you.

While every effort has been made to present a way forward for those who live with functional conditions, experts have much yet to understand. This book is a challenge to you and your healthcare providers to start a conversation, and to bring together some of the current thinking about what can cause your symptoms and what you can do to improve or even recover. If you can view your condition in a different light, it may reveal new means available to restore you to your optimal health.

This may sound strange, but many of my patients who have overcome their functional condition express gratitude for their experience. It taught them a lot that they needed to understand about themselves; it forced them to extend themselves and learn new skills and abilities that they did not know they were capable of. Most importantly, they learnt to listen to, to tend to the real needs of, and to love their dearest friend – their body.

It is my heartfelt hope that this book has helped to bring a new perspective to your condition. For the latest research in this area, you are welcome to join me on my website, where I will share ongoing information via my posts, videos and blog – www.whatthehellbook.com. While I believe that further research into functional symptoms will bring a better understanding, for now all that is left is to wish you well on your journey towards health.

Appendix A
Definitions

As you will see from the following definitions, efforts to define 'functional conditions' remain unsatisfactory. The only thing in favour of the confusing name 'functional' is that it was voted the preferred term in a survey! I have drawn on the definitions provided by Kurt Fritzsche, Susan McDaniel and Michael Wirsching (editors) in their book *Psychosomatic Medicine: An International Guide for the Primary Care Setting*. I use their terms because some of this book is based on their already well-researched and -developed therapeutic guidelines.

Medically unexplained symptoms (MUS)

'Medically unexplained symptoms' is a broad term for all the conditions where the tests cannot find a physical cause.

It is useful to divide these conditions into two categories: involuntary, where the patient has no conscious control over the symptoms, and voluntary, where the patient is consciously creating the symptoms.

Involuntary disorders

Bodily distress disorder

Bodily distress disorder is characterised by:

- the presence of bodily symptoms that are distressing to the individual
- excessive attention directed toward the symptoms, which may be manifest by repeated contact with healthcare providers.

If another health condition is causing or contributing to the symptoms, the degree of attention is clearly excessive in relation to its nature and progression.

Excessive attention is not alleviated by appropriate clinical examination and investigations and appropriate reassurance.

Bodily symptoms are persistent, being present on most days for at least several months.

Typically, bodily distress disorder involves multiple bodily symptoms that may vary over time. Occasionally there is a single symptom – usually pain or fatigue – that is associated with the other features of this disorder.

The symptoms and associated distress and preoccupation have at least some impact on the individual's functioning (for example, strain in relationships, less effective academic or occupational functioning or abandonment of specific leisure activities.)

While this latest effort to put all somatic conditions in one basket has certain advantages, there is concern that the assumption that all the syndromes under its rubric are entirely psychogenic is being challenged.

Conversion disorder

More recently called 'functional neurological disorder', a conversion disorder is a set of nervous system (neurological) symptoms that cannot be explained by a neurological disease or other medical condition. The cause is poorly understood but it relates to how the brain functions rather than any damage to the brain structure. However, the symptoms are real and cause significant distress or problems functioning. Examples would be seizures, paralysis or blindness.

Functional conditions or functional somatic symptoms

Functional conditions or functional somatic symptoms are a disturbance of normal functioning of bodily processes; these occur in a body when all the tests of the body appear normal, but the body 'misbehaves'. This term is preferred in this book, because there is not a simplistic assumption that the symptoms arise solely from the mind.

Hypochondriasis
Hypochondriasis is also called 'health anxiety'. It is characterised by an excessive degree of concern about the seriousness of even minor symptoms. Worry can lead to multiple presentations to doctors for seemingly trivial complaints, which may or may not be functional. The doctor's efforts to reassure are often met with disbelief. The conviction that something is or is about to be seriously wrong with the body can be overwhelming.

Hysteria
Hysteria is an antiquated, imprecise and very gendered term for a psychological disorder where psychological stress was converted into physical symptoms (somatisation) or a change in self-awareness such as a fugue state or selective amnesia.

Hysteria was originally applied to young women on the assumption by the ancient Egyptians that their womb (called *hystera* in Ancient Greek) would wander around the body. But lumped together under this label then were a range of conditions – from atypical migraine, epilepsy, dissociative disorders, conversion disorders, dissociative disorders and histrionic personality disorder. In other words, it is a very imprecise and lazy term that should probably be abandoned.

Organic or physical conditions
Organic or physical conditions are what we all understand as the usual health problems that have a recognisable pattern of symptoms and physical signs as well as specific tests to confirm them. Examples would be pneumonia, high blood pressure or infection.

Psychogenic symptoms
Psychogenic symptoms have a psychological cause rather than a physical one. This term will be used occasionally, but, as mentioned,

the broader contributing factors of culture, biology, genetics, epigenetics, immunology and vascular tone may also contribute to the nature of the symptom.

Psychosomatic symptoms

Psychosomatic symptoms arise from activity in the mind. With certain symptoms, such as the tears of sadness or the butterflies of fright, it is a useful and straightforward term. But for the scope of this book, it is overly simplistic, because it ignores the other bio-psychosocioimmunosexual elements that may affect the expression of psychological state.

Somatic symptom disorder

Somatic symptom disorder is the diagnostic category for functional conditions in the psychiatric classification of DSM-5, developed by the American Psychiatric Association.

Somatoform disorder

Somatoform disorder is the diagnostic category used in the previous psychiatric classification, ICD-10, the International Classification of Diseases, 10th edition. This disorder is characterised by the following features:

- repeated presentation of somatic symptoms
- persistent demand for medical attention despite the lack of any organic findings (dysfunctional illness behaviour)
- denial of emotional problems, although a close relationship exists between the somatic symptoms and psychosocial life events or conflicts (somatic fixation)
- doctor–patient relationship is characterised by disappointment and frustration.

This term has been abandoned now due to some stigmatisation around the word 'somatoform'. The preferred term now is 'bodily distress disorder', in the latest classification, ICD-11.

Somatisation

Somatisation is a psychological problem or emotional disorder expressed somatically or in a bodily symptom. It refers to the tendency of a person to have physical symptoms in response to stress or emotions. So, for example, if you get a headache when under pressure, you might be said to be somatising or to be a somatiser. But somatisation does not necessarily lead to a somatic symptom disorder.

Stress

Stress is broadly defined as a response to a perceived threat, danger, excessive demand or other stimuli (stressor).

Stressor

Stressors are what trigger a stress response. Stressors can be physical, financial, emotional, psychological, immunological, genetic, epigenetic, social or existential.

Voluntary disorders

While these disorders are not dealt with in this book, I've included definitions for them here for completeness and to make the strong distinction between deliberate and deceptive behaviour and other functional conditions. It is critical to exclude these two conditions before therapy can be considered for the involuntary functional disorders.

Factitious disorder

Factitious disorder is a serious mental disorder in which someone deceives others by appearing to be sick, by purposely getting sick or by self-injury. The reason for this behaviour is poorly understood. Seeking the sick role and consequent medical attention appears to be the purpose.

Malingering

The behaviour of the malingerer is similar to those with factitious disorder, but the motive is for personal gain – for example, a soldier injuring himself to get out of active service or to make a compensation claim.

Appendix B

The seven body stress systems

The following figures outline the seven body stress systems, the factors that disrupt them and the resulting symptoms. (Refer to chapter 4 for more information on these systems and potential symptoms.)

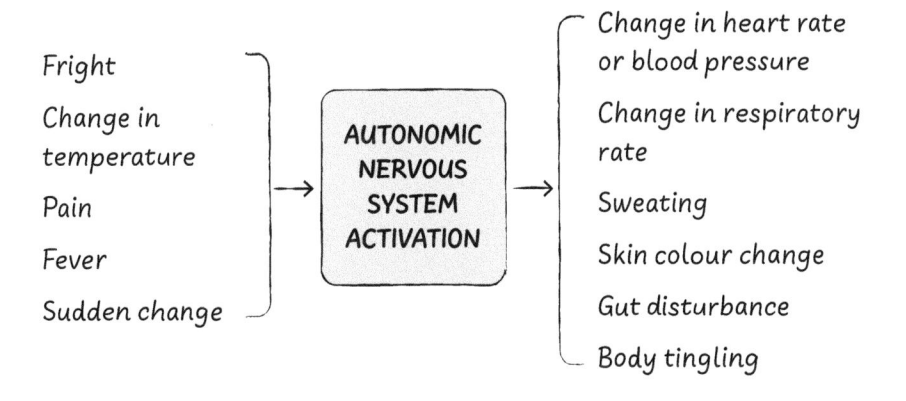

Autonomic nervous system

Fright
Change in temperature
Pain
Fever
Sudden change

→ **AUTONOMIC NERVOUS SYSTEM ACTIVATION** →

Change in heart rate or blood pressure
Change in respiratory rate
Sweating
Skin colour change
Gut disturbance
Body tingling

The hormone system and hypothalamic–pituitary–adrenal axis

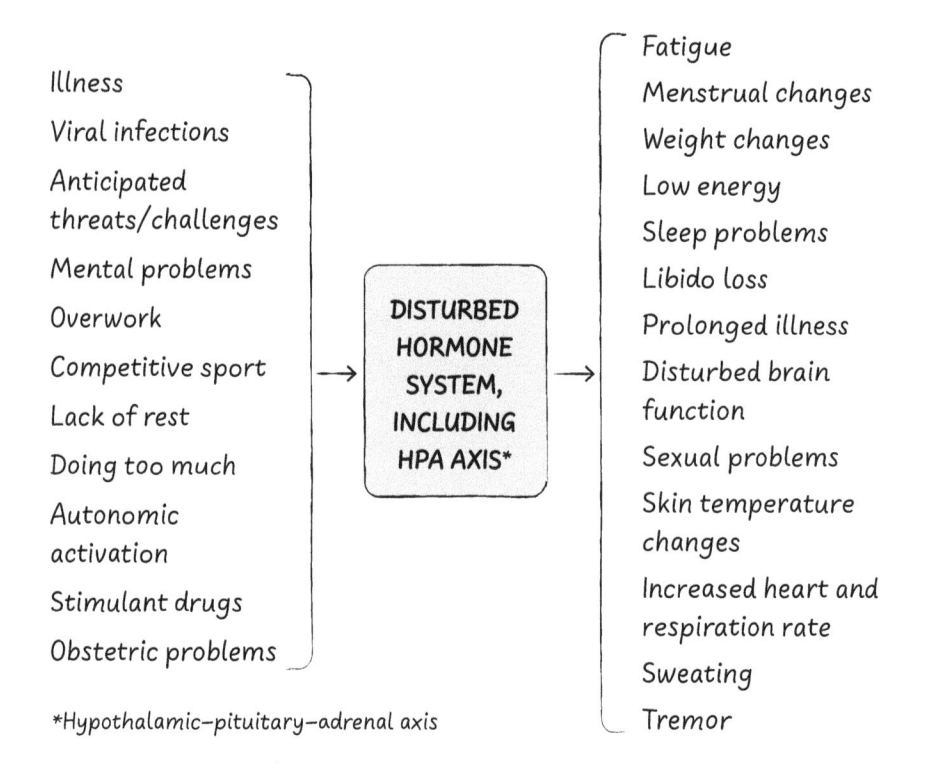

Inputs:
- Illness
- Viral infections
- Anticipated threats/challenges
- Mental problems
- Overwork
- Competitive sport
- Lack of rest
- Doing too much
- Autonomic activation
- Stimulant drugs
- Obstetric problems

→ **DISTURBED HORMONE SYSTEM, INCLUDING HPA AXIS*** →

Outputs:
- Fatigue
- Menstrual changes
- Weight changes
- Low energy
- Sleep problems
- Libido loss
- Prolonged illness
- Disturbed brain function
- Sexual problems
- Skin temperature changes
- Increased heart and respiration rate
- Sweating
- Tremor

*Hypothalamic–pituitary–adrenal axis

Immune-inflammatory system

Inputs:
- Illness
- Poor nutrition
- Vaccination
- Genetics
- Epigenetics
- Stress
- Anxiety
- Depression
- Trauma

→ **DISRUPTION TO IMMUNE-INFLAMMATORY SYSTEM** →

Outputs:
- Rashes
- Swelling
- Aches and pains
- Severe reaction to illness
- Colitis
- Dyshidrotic eczema
- Prostatitis
- Anal itch

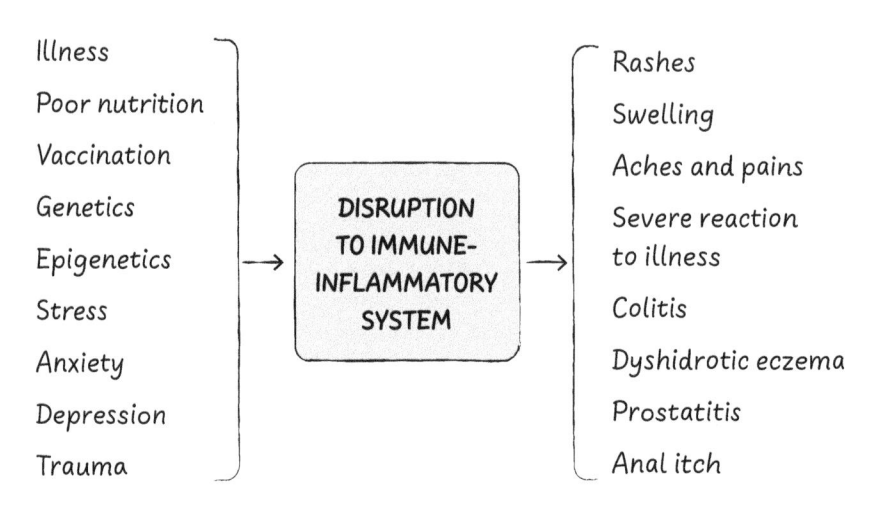

THE SEVEN BODY STRESS SYSTEMS

Circadian rhythm

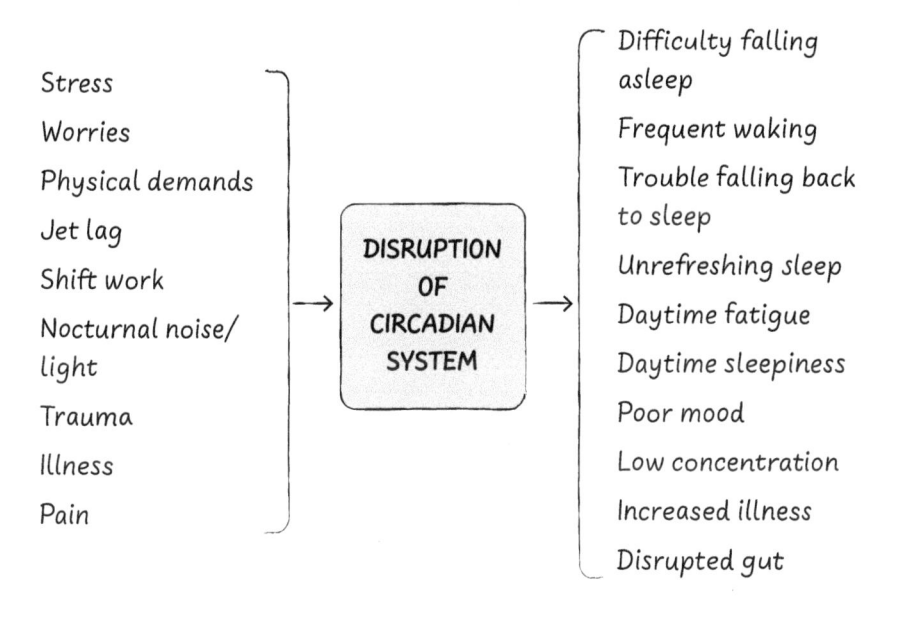

Stress
Worries
Physical demands
Jet lag
Shift work
Nocturnal noise/light
Trauma
Illness
Pain

→ **DISRUPTION OF CIRCADIAN SYSTEM** →

Difficulty falling asleep
Frequent waking
Trouble falling back to sleep
Unrefreshing sleep
Daytime fatigue
Daytime sleepiness
Poor mood
Low concentration
Increased illness
Disrupted gut

Skeletomotor system

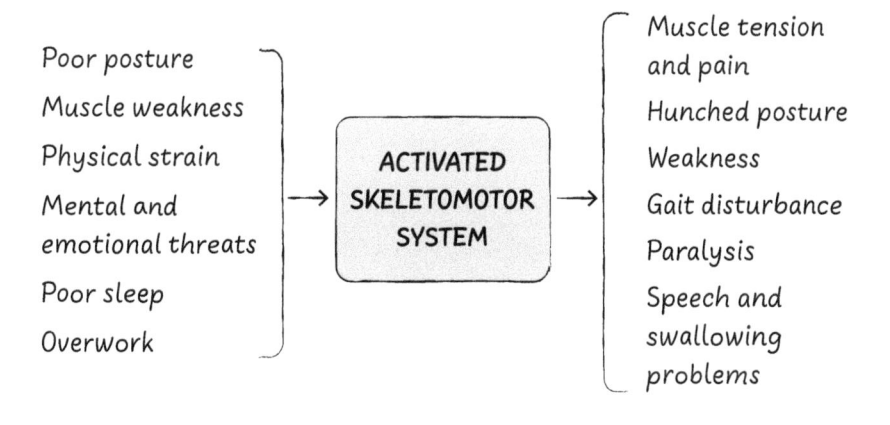

Poor posture
Muscle weakness
Physical strain
Mental and emotional threats
Poor sleep
Overwork

→ **ACTIVATED SKELETOMOTOR SYSTEM** →

Muscle tension and pain
Hunched posture
Weakness
Gait disturbance
Paralysis
Speech and swallowing problems

Microbiota–gut–brain system

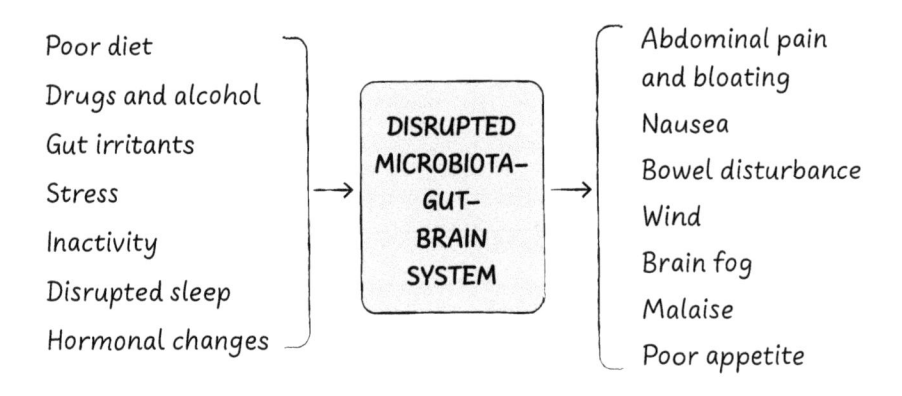

Poor diet
Drugs and alcohol
Gut irritants
Stress
Inactivity
Disrupted sleep
Hormonal changes

→ **DISRUPTED MICROBIOTA–GUT–BRAIN SYSTEM** →

Abdominal pain and bloating
Nausea
Bowel disturbance
Wind
Brain fog
Malaise
Poor appetite

Brain stress system

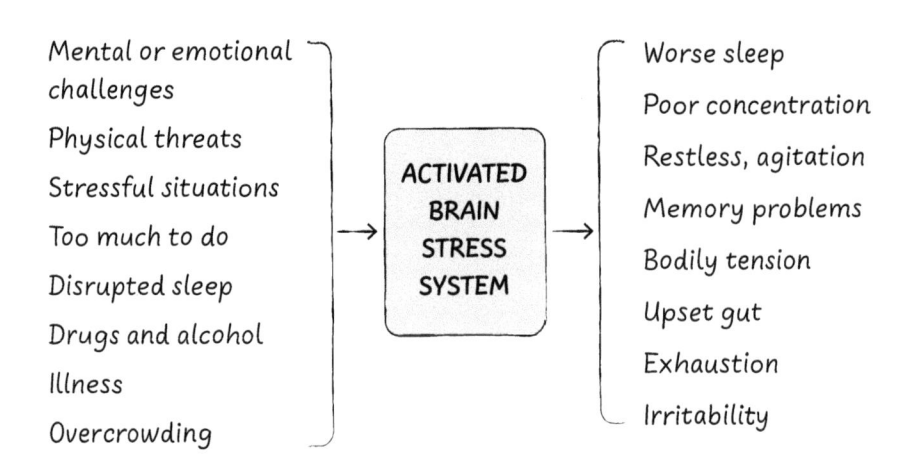

Mental or emotional challenges
Physical threats
Stressful situations
Too much to do
Disrupted sleep
Drugs and alcohol
Illness
Overcrowding

→ **ACTIVATED BRAIN STRESS SYSTEM** →

Worse sleep
Poor concentration
Restless, agitation
Memory problems
Bodily tension
Upset gut
Exhaustion
Irritability

Appendix C

Useful resources

BeyondBlue – mental health information and support www.beyondblue.org.au.

Black Dog Institute – for mental health resources: www.blackdoginstitute.org.au/resources-support/digital-tools-apps.

Blue Knot Foundation – useful resource on trauma and abuse, providing support and tools, and help via the National Redress Scheme for survivors of institutional child sexual abuse: www.blueknot.org.au.

Butterfly Foundation – offering understanding that everyone's experience of an eating disorder or body image issue is unique, and access to effective services: www.butterfly.org.au.

Fibromyalgia Australia – patient information for fibromyalgia: www.fibromyalgiaaustralia.org.au.

FND Australia Support Services – support for those with Functional Neurological Disorder. FND Australia Support Services, including a 12 week course on FND wellbeing. www.FNDAus.org.au

FND Hope – an excellent resource for those with functional neurological disorders: www.fndhope.org.

For Professionals: Functional Somatic Symptoms in Children and Adolescents: a Stress System Approach to Assessment and Treatment by Professor Kasia Kozlowska, Stephen Scher, Helene Helgeland.

IBS Central, Monash University – information about irritable bowel syndrome and how to treat it: www.monashfodmap.com/ibs-central.

Migraine and Headache Australia – a good source of information and treatment options: www.headacheaustralia.org.au.

Overeaters Anonymous – a community of people who support each other in order to recover from compulsive eating and food behaviours, welcoming everyone who feels they have a problem with food: www.oa.org.

Professor Lorimer Moseley (neuroscientist and founder of charity Painrevolution) has developed some wonderful material that provides easily accessible information and resources to help you learn conditions:

- www.painrevolution.org – should be essential reading for all who experience ongoing pain
- 'Why things hurt', TEDxAdelaide – keep watching this until you understand what he is saying, it may help: www.youtube.com/watch?v=gwd-wLdIHjs.
- 'Pain, the brain and your amazing protectometer', Musculoskeletal Australia – definitely watch this if you want to understand pain: www.youtube.com/watch?v=lCF1_Fs00nM&t=1011s.

'Sleep hygiene', Better Health Channel – tips on how to improve your sleep: www.betterhealth.vic.gov.au/health/conditionsandtreatments/sleep-hygiene.

The Australian and New Zealand Headache Society – The Australian and New Zealand Headache Society (ANZHS) website, www.anzheadachesociety.org, provides resources for healthcare professionals, researchers and patients on headache disorders. It offers access to research, clinical guidelines, and educational materials, aiming to improve patient care and foster specialist collaboration. The site also details upcoming conferences, events, and membership opportunities.

'This talk may cause side effects', Festival of Dangerous Ideas – Dr Kate Faasse's brilliant expose about the nocebo effect and the problem with informed consent: www.events.unsw.edu.au/article/this-talk-may-cause-side-effects-kate-faasse.

Appendix D

Illness behaviour questionnaire

The questions provided here can help to shape your understanding of your response to illness. Remember – these questions don't have a right or wrong answer, but rather can help you shape your understanding of how your symptoms are affecting you and what could be different.

These are the sort of questions your psychologist or counsellor would like to know the answers to. And your answers may prompt you to open a discussion about them with family and loved ones.

Do you worry a lot about your health?	YES	NO
Do you think there is something seriously wrong with your body?	YES	NO
Does your illness interfere with your life a great deal?	YES	NO
Are you easiest to get along with when you are ill?	YES	NO
Does your family have a history of illness?	YES	NO
Do you think you are more liable to illness than other people?	YES	NO
If doctors told you that they could find nothing wrong with you, would you believe them?	YES	NO
Is it easy for you to forget about yourself and think about all sorts of other things?	YES	NO

If you feel ill and someone tells you that you are looking better, do you become annoyed?	YES	NO
Do you find that you are often aware of various things happening in your body?	YES	NO
Do you ever think of your illness as a punishment for something you have done wrong in the past?	YES	NO
Do you have trouble with your nerves?	YES	NO
If you feel ill or worried, can you be easily cheered up by the doctor?	YES	NO
Do you think that other people realise what it is like to be sick?	YES	NO
Does it upset you to talk to the doctor about your illness?	YES	NO
Are you bothered by many pains and aches?	YES	NO
Does your illness affect the way you get along with your family or friends a great deal?	YES	NO
Do you find that you get anxious easily?	YES	NO
Do you know anybody who has had the same illness as you?	YES	NO
Are you more sensitive to pain than other people?	YES	NO
Are you afraid of illness?	YES	NO
Can you express your personal feelings easily to other people?	YES	NO
Do people feel sorry for you when you are ill?	YES	NO
Do you think that you worry about your health more than most people?	YES	NO
Do you find that your illness affects your sexual relations?	YES	NO
Do you experience a lot of pain with your illness?	YES	NO
Except for your illness, do you have any problems in your life?	YES	NO

ILLNESS BEHAVIOUR QUESTIONNAIRE

Do you care whether or not people realise you are sick?	YES	NO
Do you find that you get jealous of other people's good health?	YES	NO
Do you ever have silly thoughts about your health that you can't get out of your mind, no matter how hard you try?	YES	NO
Do you have any financial problems?	YES	NO
Are you upset by the way people take your illness?	YES	NO
Is it hard for you to believe doctors when they tell you there is nothing for you to worry about?	YES	NO
Do you often worry about the possibility that you have got a serious illness?	YES	NO
Are you sleeping well?	YES	NO
When you are angry, do you tend to bottle up your feelings?	YES	NO
Do you often think that you might suddenly fall ill?	YES	NO
If a disease is brought to your attention (through the radio, television, newspapers or someone you know) do you worry about getting it yourself?	YES	NO
Do you get the feeling that people are not taking your illness seriously enough?	YES	NO
Are you upset by the appearance of your face or body?	YES	NO
Do you find that you are bothered by many different symptoms?	YES	NO
Do you frequently try to explain to others how you are feeling?	YES	NO
Do you have any family problems?	YES	NO
Do you think there is something the matter with your mind?	YES	NO
Are you eating well?	YES	NO

Is your bad health the biggest difficulty of your life?	YES	NO
Do you find that you get sad easily?	YES	NO
Do you worry or fuss over small details that seem unimportant to others?	YES	NO
Are you always a co-operative patient?	YES	NO
Do you often have the symptoms of a very serious disease?	YES	NO
Do you find that you get angry easily?	YES	NO
Do you have any work problems?	YES	NO
Do you prefer to keep your feelings to yourself?	YES	NO
Do you often find that you get depressed?	YES	NO
Would all your worries be over if you were physically healthy?	YES	NO
Are you more irritable towards other people?	YES	NO
Do you think that your symptoms may be caused by worry?	YES	NO
Is it easy for you to let people know when you are cross with them?	YES	NO
Is it hard for you to relax?	YES	NO
Do you have personal worries which are not caused by physical illness?	YES	NO
Do you often find that you lose patience with other people?	YES	NO
Is it hard for you to show people your personal feelings?	YES	NO

Index

A

abdominal breathing 184
abdominal pain 2, 27, 30, 55, 94
accelerated heart rate 26
acute pain 79–82
addressing doubts 147
'air hunger' 26, 49, 50
alcohol 75, 105, 156
allergies 60
anxiety 26, 55, 105–106, 129, 150, 214
aquarobics 197–198
autonomic nervous system 42, 45–51, 136, 225
—environment and 181–184
avoidance 203–204
Ayurvedic medicine 103

B

back pain 26, 29, 91–92, 128, 146
'Bermuda Triangle of medicine' 16
biopsychosocial model 125–126
bloating 30
blood flow 48
blushing 26, 48
bodily distress disorder 219–220
body stress systems 6, 14, 39–76, 146–150, 153–158, 225–228
—restoring 181–208
body temperature 36–37, 50
bottom-up approach 167–171
box breathing 184
brain–body connection 6, 36–44
brain fog 27, 111
brain stress system 71–74, 228
brain system 43, 137, 200–207
breast pain 95
breathing difficulties 26, 49–50, 55, 183–184
breathwork 183–184
broken heart syndrome 58
building your team 165–179
burnout 104–105, 202
'butterflies' in the stomach 24

C

cardiovascular system 48
chest pain 2, 19, 23, 26, 54, 55, 57, 93, 94
chest tightness 29, 50, 55
childhood trauma 29, 55, 178, 185
chills 27, 55, 128
'chronic' illness 21
chronic pain 79–82
circadian rhythm 43, 63–66, 137, 190–193, 214, 227
clearing the air 176–178
collapsed immobility 74
collapsing 2, 31–32, 118
complex regional pain syndrome 86–88
concentration problems 109–111
conscious activity 43–44, 53, 90
constipation 26, 64
contagiousness 24
conversion disorder 220
cortisol levels 110, 185
coughing 2, 24
COVID-19 59, 104, 108, 120

cramps 27, 30, 50, 116
craniosacral therapy 169
crying 23, 27, 50

D

Darwin, Charles 45–46
defensive mode 36–39, 45, 49, 59, 62, 72, 110, 148–149, 185, 201–202
depression 105–106, 118, 214
diagnosis 5, 18, 141–144, 157–158
— importance of 20
diet 102–103, 198–200
digestion 26, 48, 51, 74, 188
disease versus illness 124–127
disorders 28, 210
dissociation 73
dizziness 24, 27, 55, 92
doctor–patient relationship 159–163
dry mouth 26, 56
dyspepsia 26

E

ear pain 93
eczema 60
eight-hour days 104–106
emotions 24, 27, 48, 50
Engel, Dr George 125–127
epigenetics 41–42, 130
epilepsy 147, 177, 214
erectile dysfunction 26, 53–54
exercise 51, 62, 68, 153, 194–198
— graded approach to 196–197
exhaustion 99–112
expectancy effect 116–117

F

Faasse, Dr Kate 118–119
factitious disorder 223
faintness 2, 24, 32, 27, 50
'faking it' 13–16
fasting 102–103
fatigue 6, 27, 99–112, 128
— defining 99–101
— mental health and 105–106

fear 48
— of dying 27, 55
— of going mad 27, 55
feeling of dread 26, 55, 178
feeling of unreality 27, 50, 56
fever 128
fibromyalgia 28, 96–97
fight, flight or freeze 37, 51, 73–74
fleeting pain 27
'fullness of the brain' 50
functional neurological disorder 220
functional symptoms 2
— causes of 7–8, 35–44, 207
— definition of 6, 11–12, 17–18, 23–33, 35

G

gait disturbance 27, 67–68
genetics 5, 40–42, 130
Gilbert syndrome 133
'glitch in your software' 12–13
globus 30, 210
glucocorticoid use 128
green flags 131–132
grief 31
Gupta Program 170
gut disturbances 6, 27, 69–70, 214

H

headaches 25–26, 29, 90–91, 127, 212
head fog 50
healthcare providers 165–167
healthcare team 6
hearing problems 27
heart palpitations 168, 178
'heartsink' patients 205–207
heaviness 24
hives 60
homeostasis 36
hope 171–172
hormone system 42–43, 51–59, 136, 187–188, 226
hot flushes 27, 55
hydrotherapy 197–198

INDEX

hyperhidrosis 27, 210
hyperventilation 50, 56, 111
hypochondriasis 221
hypothalamic-pituitary-adrenal system 42–43, 51–59, 226
— restoring 185–188
hypothalamus 53–55
hysteria 221

I

illness
— culture and 16
— history of 16–18
illness behaviours 14, 129, 176, 233–236
immune-inflammatory system 43, 59–66, 137, 188–190, 226
inability to move 24
incontinence 27
indigestion 26
inflammation 27
'informed' consent 120–121
involuntary nervous system *see* autonomic nervous system
irregular bowel actions 30
irritable bowel syndrome 27, 30–31, 212

J

joint pain 27

K

karoshi 202
Kozlowska, Prof. Kasia 4, 62, 150, 191

L

life expectancy 15, 37
lightheadedness 27, 55
loss of consciousness 1, 27, 50
lump in the throat 27, 29–30

M

macrophages 61–63
malingering 13, 224
massage 153, 166, 182
mass reactions 24–25
medical history 155, 160
'medically unexplained symptoms' 11
medical system 123–137
medication 213–214
Mediterranean diet 199
melatonin 214
memory problems 109–111
menopause 53, 156–157, 187
menstrual cycle 51, 53
mental health 205–207, 214
microbiome-gut-brain system 43, 69–70, 137, 198–200, 228
modern medicine 5, 6, 17
morphine 113–117
Moseley, Prof. Lorimer 55
muscle pain 27, 59, 119–120
muscle weakness 177
myofascial pain syndrome 96

N

nature versus nurture 40–42
nausea 2, 24, 27, 40, 55, 64, 120–121
negative thoughts 113–122
neural pathways 20
neuroplasticity 204–205
nocebo effect 113–122
'normal' test results 5, 12, 15, 18–20, 54, 57, 58, 161
numbness 24, 27, 49, 50

O

osteoporosis 128
overwork 202

P

pain 1, 6, 24, 79–97, 128
panic attacks 54–58, 89, 166, 168, 178, 185
— causes of 56
pelvic pain 95–96
personal sanctuary 182–183
placebo effect 114–117

postural orthostatic tachycardia syndrome 58–59, 186–187
predictive processing model 88–90
psychogenic symptoms 221–222
psychologists 173–179
psychoneuroendoimmunology 63
'psychosomatic' response 48, 222

Q
qi gong 169
quality of life 15

R
radiculopathy 128
rapid heart rate 39, 50, 54, 55
rashes 6, 17, 27
Red Flag method 91
red flags 127–129
reductionism 124–125
referred pain 93–94
reflux 29, 30, 193
repetitive strain injury 86–88
restorative mode 37–39, 45, 49, 59, 62, 150, 201–202
rigid muscles 50
risk factors 142

S
seizures 1, 24
self-efficacy 175–176
sexual functioning 51, 187
sexual trauma 173–174
shaking 27, 55
'shell shock' 74
side effects of medication 118–121
skeletomotor system 43, 66–68, 137, 193–198, 227
skin problems 60
sleep 102, 110, 190–193
 — problems with 39, 63, 101–102
smoking 75
somatic nervous system 46
somatic symptom disorder 222

somatisation 223
somatoform disorder 222
sore throat 6
specialists 1, 7, 30, 55, 132, 158
speech problems 1, 27, 30
statins 119–120
stiffness 128
stress 6, 15, 20, 24, 35, 40, 45–76, 129, 150, 177, 223
 — 'invention of' 44
stress response system 83
subconscious activity 44, 47, 53, 54, 90
swallowing disorders 27
sweating 24, 27, 41, 50, 55
swelling 27
swimming 197–198
symptoms 1–2, 5–6, 28, 37–38, 146, 154–156, 209
 — enduring 57
 — intermittent 6
 — managing 8
 — persistence of 1, 15
syndromes 28, 209

T
takotsubo cardiomyopathy 58, 214
tension headaches 25–26
threats 47
tingling 14, 27, 50, 55
tinnitus 27
tonic immobility 74
top-down approach 167–171
traditional versus functional medical history taking 155
trauma-informed therapy 163, 185–186
treatment options 145–152, 209–215
trembling 27, 55
trust 162–163
twitches 27

U

unconsciousness 24
undiagnosed illness 1, 108, 160
urination problems 27, 95

V

vision problems 24, 26, 27, 50
vital signs 17
voluntary nervous system
   see somatic nervous system

W

walking difficulties 2
'watchful expectation' 100
weakness 1, 27
weight gain 108, 177, 178, 199
weight loss 128
whiplash 92–93

Y

yellow flags 129–130, 177
Yerkes-Dodson curve 201, 204

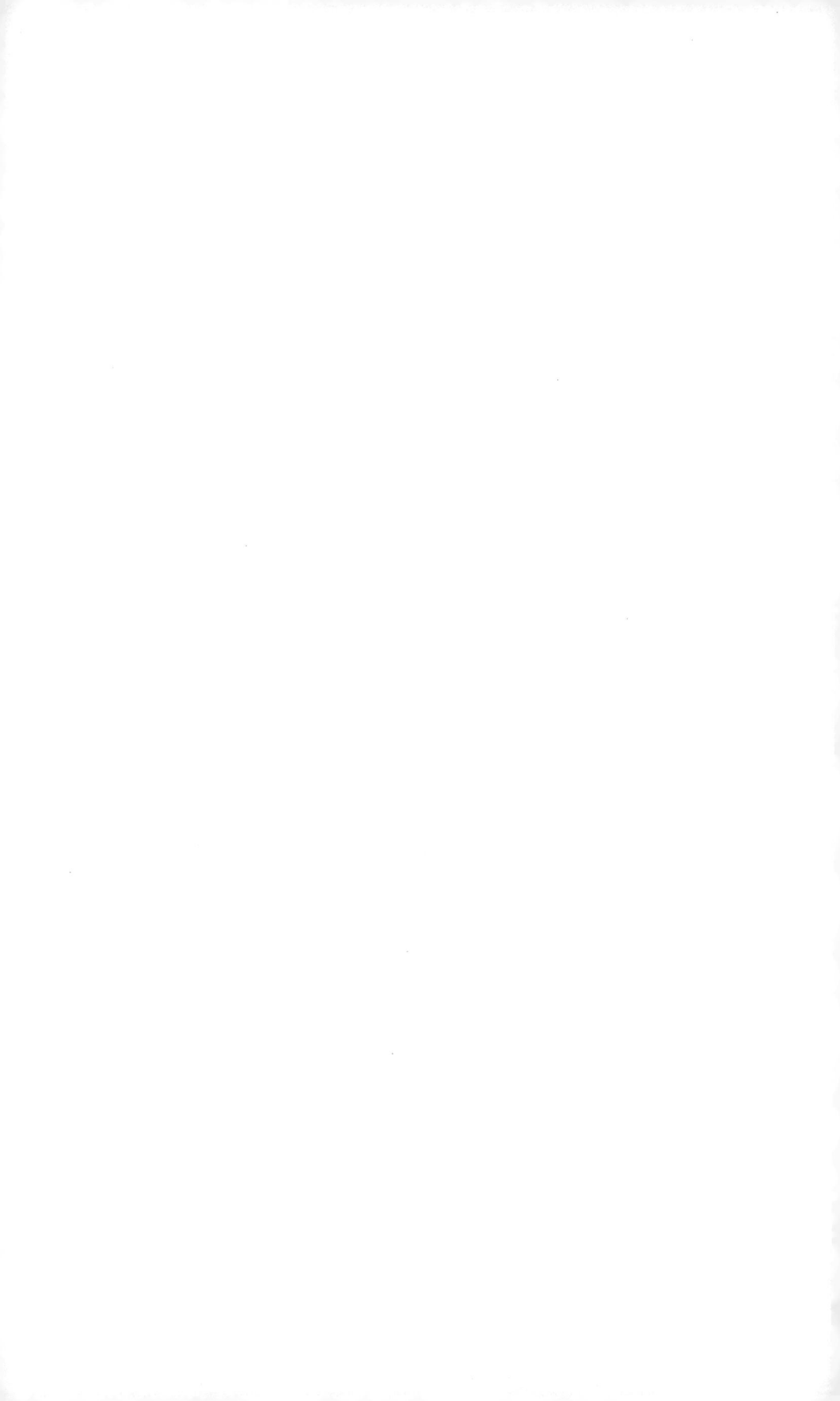